Healthy and Easy Recipes For Al

This recipe book has been created to help everyone eat more nutrient-d... that makes you feel good.

All recipes are **vegan** and **gluten-free** but this book is not just for people following those diets.

Whether you are vegan, health conscious, allergic to dairy or just trying to incorporate some more healthy plant-based recipes into your diet you will find something here.

Healthy

This is not a low-calorie recipe book, but it is a **no empty calorie** recipe book. All recipes are nutrient-dense, high in vitamins and minerals.

Recipes don't contain refined ingredients such as white flour and sugar that are empty calories. Many do contain a sweetener like dates or maple syrup. These natural sweeteners are not just pure refined sugar (although they are high in sugar) and contain some vitamins and minerals.

If you are following a low sugar diet you can reduce or change the amount of fruit or sweetener in these recipes.

Easy

There's no difficulty level for recipes as all are easy. Some may have long lists of ingredients (like the chocolate brownie) and many steps but they are still easy and almost foolproof to make.

Recipe Key

Nut Free
nf
Free of tree nuts and peanuts

Raw
raw
Not heated and contains ingredients generally accepted on a raw food diet

Paleo
p
Suitable for a palaeolithic diet, free of legumes, grains and pseudo grains

Oil-free
Nothing is fried with oil. Some recipes do contain a small amount of oil and this is optional or can be substituted. See "Coconut Butter" on page 10 and see "Oil Free Adaptations" on page 24.

Gluten-free
All recipes are gluten-free, some contain oats so buy Gluten free oats if you are sensitive to gluten, see "Oats and Gluten" on page 80.

Grain-free
Most recipes are grain-free however some do contain oats. The pseudo grains Quinoa (page 4) and Buckwheat (page 20) are used extensively.

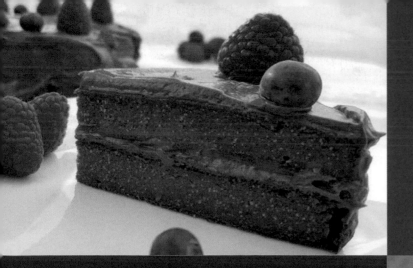

Cakes 4

Candy & Fudge 26

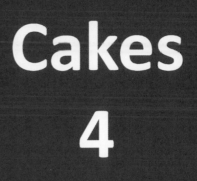

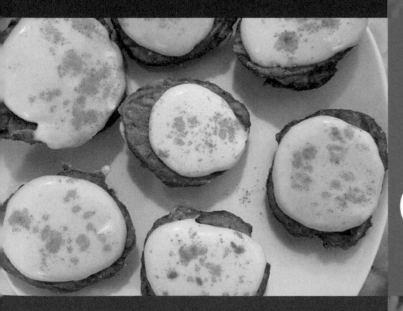

Baked Goodies 54

Desserts 70

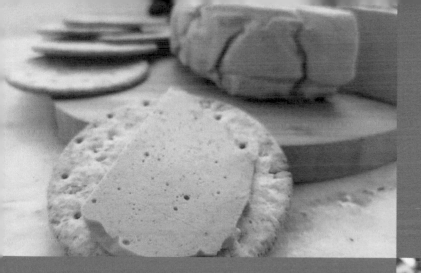

Sides
94

Snacks
118

Mains
142

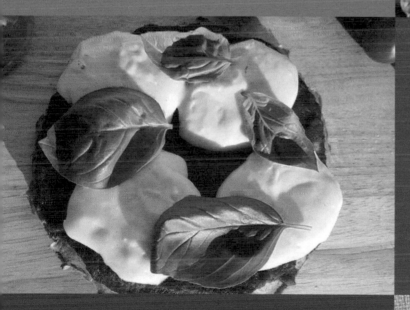

Drinks
172

Quinoa Avocado Chocolate Fudge Cake

Makes 8 servings | 1h 20 mins

This Quinoa Avocado chocolate fudge healthy cake is always popular with everyone. If you're cooking it for a sceptic just call it chocolate fudge cake, they may guess it's gluten-free as it's heavier than a traditional cake but they are unlikely to guess that it's bursting with nutrition.

Quinoa Chocolate Cake

- 1½ cups / 250g **Quinoa**
- 2 cups / 450ml **Water**
- 1 cup / 175g **Dates**, pitted
- 1 tsp **Vanilla**
- 1 tsp **Baking powder**
- 4 tbsp **Cocoa powder**
- 2 tbsp **Chia seeds**
- a pinch of **Salt**
- 2-4 tbsp **Sweetener** such as Maple syrup

Avocado Chocolate Icing (raw)

- 2 **Avocados**
- 4-6 tbsp **Sweetener** such as Maple syrup
- 2 tbsp **Coconut oil / butter**, you can leave out but the icing won't set as firm
- 4 tbsp **Cacao / Cocoa powder**

Fruit for decoration, like **bright berries**

Equipment

- Food processor / blender
- 2 Cake tins 6" and Oven

Method

1. Soak the quinoa for at least 15 minutes, then drain. Soaking for an hour or overnight is preferable.
2. Add everything else for the cake into the blender and blend until smooth.
3. Split into two lined 6" pans and bake for 35-45 minutes at 350F / 180C .
4. You can tell when it's cooked as knife comes out clean.
5. Leave to cool for 15 minutes before taking out of the pan.
6. Blend all of the icing ingredients together.
7. Ice the top of one cake, place the other cake on top then ice the top and sides.
8. Decorate with berries, store in the fridge and enjoy within 3 days.

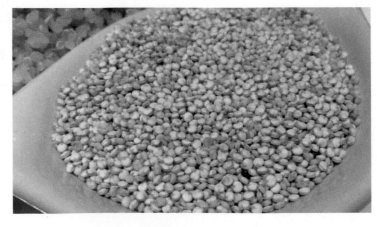

Quinoa

Quinoa is used extensively in this book as it's versatile and a handy wheat replacement.

This South American seed is used like a grain but is gluten-free and in the same family as beets and spinach.

It has twice the protein of rice and contains all nine essential amino acids.

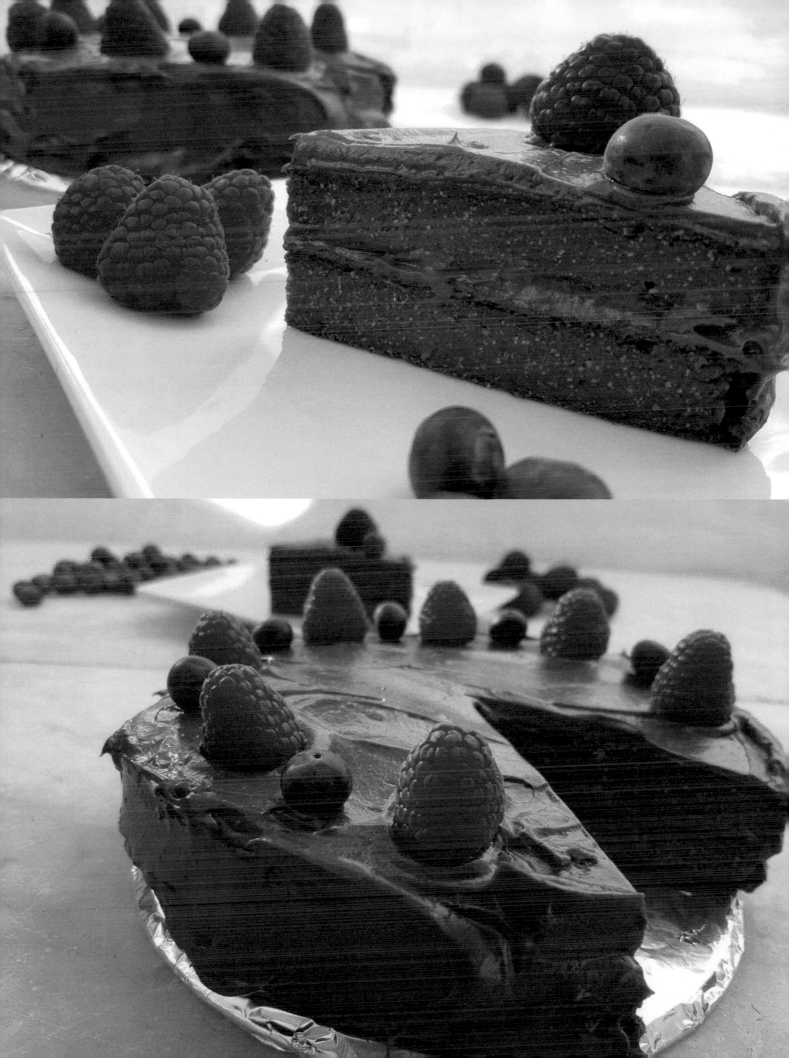

Carrot Cake Truffles with Vanilla Bean Icing

Makes 16 truffles | 25 mins (raw)

Out of all the sweets in this book this is the one I come back to the most. It's hard to beat a raw carrot cake with vanilla icing and a dash of cinnamon.

Truffles

- 2 cups / 100g **Carrot**, grated
- 1 cup / 150g **Walnuts**
- 1 cup / 175g **Dates**
- 3 tbsp **Buckwheat**
- 2 tbsp shredded **Coconut**
- 1 tbsp **Chia seeds**
- 1 tsp **Cinnamon**
- ½ tsp ground **Ginger**
- ¼ tsp **Nutmeg**

Vanilla Icing

- 1 cup / 150g **Cashews**
- ½ cup / 120ml **Coconut Butter (page 10)** or **oil**
- 3 tbsp **Maple syrup** or sweetener
- 1 tsp **Vanilla**
- 1 **Lime** juiced

Equipment

- Blender / Food processor & Double boiler
- Non-stick sheets / Cake pan & Fork

Method

1. Put all of the truffle ingredients into a food processor and pulse blend until all combined.
2. Either roll into balls for truffles and place on non stick sheets or push into a cake pan for one big carrot cake. Place in the freezer to chill while you make the icing.
3. Melt the coconut butter or oil as it is solid at a room temperature. I melt it by placing in a bowl within a pan of hot water or by using a double boiler.
4. Place all of the icing ingredients into a blender with a few tablespoons of water. Blend until you get a smooth creamy icing.
5. Hold the truffles on a fork over the icing and spoon on the cashew vanilla bean icing. Then sprinkle with cinnamon and put on a non stick sheet.
6. For the cake just pour the icing on top and spread it out. Sprinkle with cinnamon / grated carrots or chopped nuts to garnish.
7. Once the truffles / cake is made chill in the fridge for half an hour and they are ready to eat.
8. They will last several days stored in the fridge.

Raw Food Diet

I call these raw although several ingredients have been heated above 40C such as the maple syrup and cashews. Maple syrup is usually accepted on the raw food diet. Truly raw cashews are difficult to find but non roasted "raw" varieties are generally accepted. Even the ones labelled raw have almost always been steamed and lightly baked during the processing. Omit the buckwheat to make this paleo.

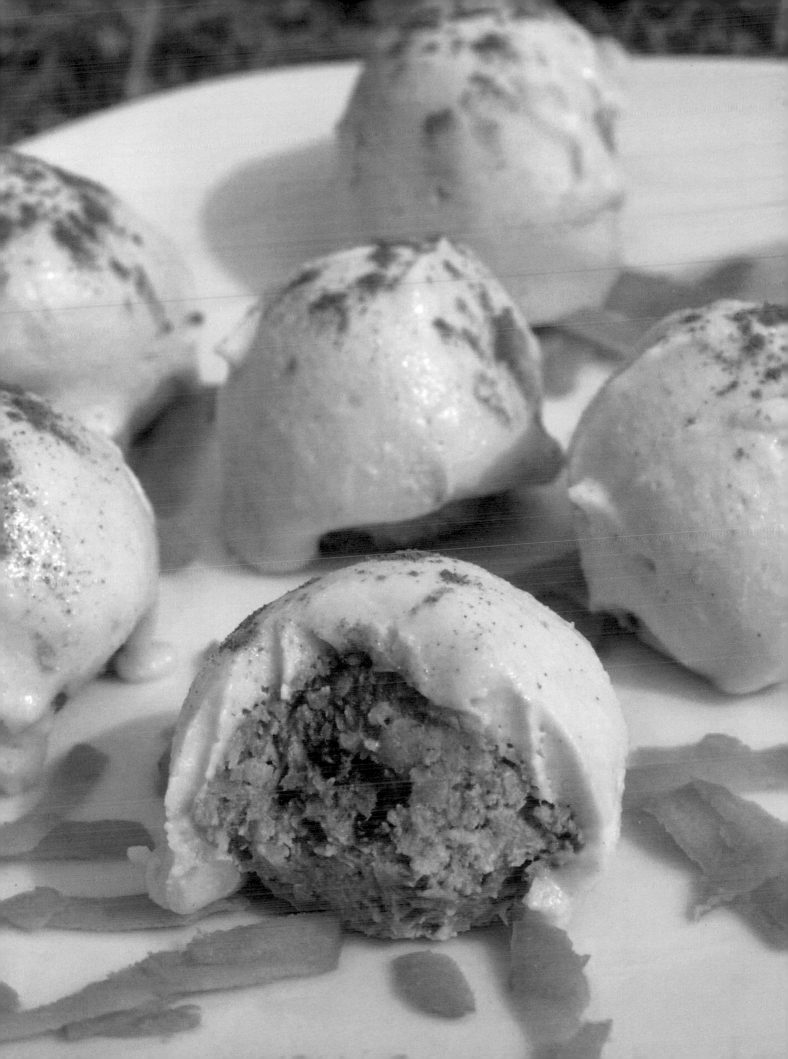

Cotton Candy Cashew Cheesecake

Serves 12 | 45 mins **raw** **p**

All the colourings are natural, organic and healthy. The ingredient list may look daunting but only the base and cashew cream ingredients are mandatory – you can use whatever fruit / berries you want for colour and flavour.

Base
- 1 cup / 175g **Dates**
- 1 cup / 125g **Walnuts**
- ½ cup / 50g **Coconut**, desiccated

Cashew cream
- 1½ cups / 225g **Cashew nuts**
- 5 tbsp **Maple syrup** / any sweetener
- 2 tsp **Vanilla** extract
- 2 **Lemons** juiced
- ½ cup / 120ml **Coconut butter/oil,** melted
- 1 cup / 240ml **Water**

To colour the cream
- ½ **Pomegranate**, juiced
- a pinch **Baking powder**
- ⅓ **Red cabbage**, juiced
- 1 cup / 100g **Blueberries**

Toppings
- **Blueberries / pomegranate seeds / any fruit**

Equipment
- Blender or Food processor
- Cake tin or Pan about 8"
- Sieve and 5 Bowls

Method
1. Blend all of the base ingredients until they stick together in a ball.
2. Push the base into a 8" pan.
3. Blend the cabbage and pomegranate and then push through a sieve to strain and make juice.
4. Separate half of the red cabbage juice and stir in the baking powder to make the blue.
5. Place all the cashew cream ingredients in a blender and whiz until smooth, remember to melt the coconut oil / butter first.
6. Separate the cream into 5 bowls.
7. Keep one bowl white, stir in 1-2 tbsp of red and blue into two other bowls.
8. In one bowl stir in 3-4 tbsp of pomegranate juice.
9. In a blender whizz together the last bowl with the blueberries.
10. Layer on the different coloured creams in the pan however you like, I did one colour at a time.
11. Place in the fridge for an hour to set.
12. Store in the fridge and enjoy within a couple of days

Notes

You don't taste the cabbage juice in this, no one has ever guessed it without being told. But if you are worried just add a drop at a time and taste it.

Half of the cashews can be replaced with Buckwheat (page 20) for a less nut-heavy cake.

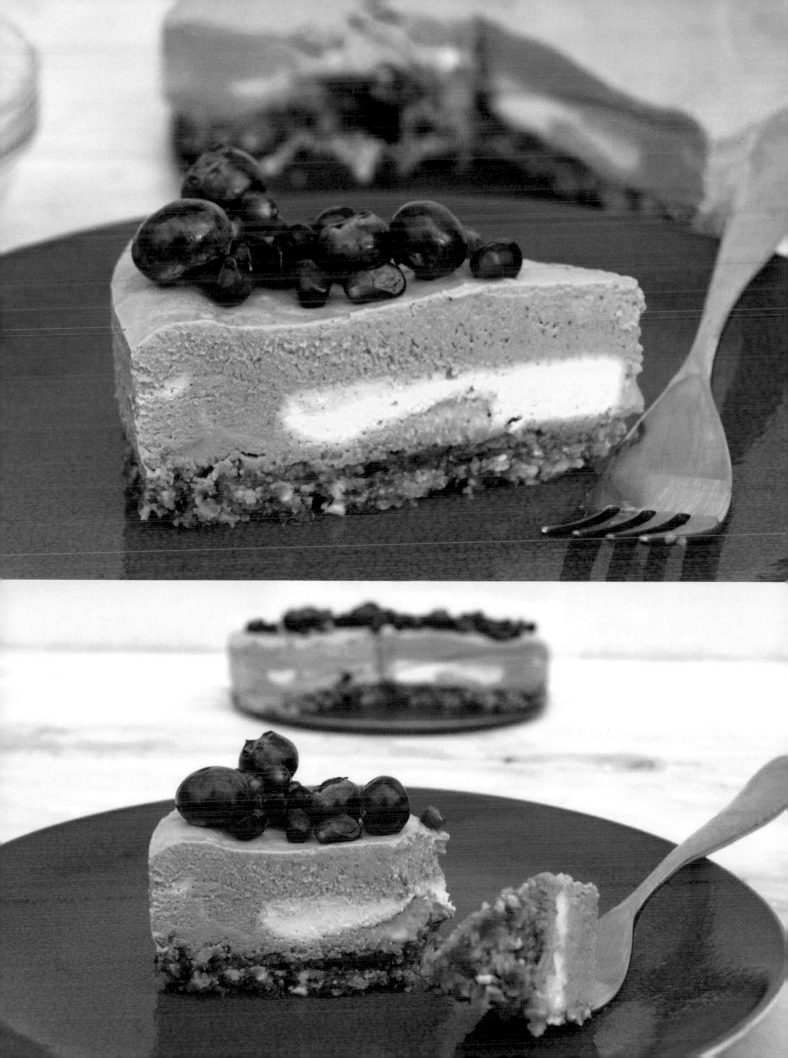

Raw Chocolate Orange Frosted Brownies

Makes 12 brownies | 20 mins

The chocolate orange flavour works really well with raw cacao and the icing tastes just as good as it looks. The only downside is that it's a bit sticky and best eaten with cutlery. Don't worry about tasting the turmeric as it's just there for colour but does also up the nutrition.

Chocolate Orange Brownies

- 1 ⅓ cups / 180g **Walnuts**
- 1 cup / 175g **Dates**
- 5 tbsp **Cacao / Cocoa**
- 3 tbsp **Chia seeds**
- 1 **Orange**, juiced

Equipment

- Blender / food processor and 8" pan

Orange Cashew Frosting

- 1 cup / 150g **Cashew nuts**
- 3 tbsp **Coconut butter / oil,** melted
- 2 tbsp **Maple syrup**
- 1 **Orange**, juiced
- 1 tsp **Vanilla**
- ¼ tsp **Turmeric**
- 2 tsp **Orange zest**

Method

1. Place everything for the brownie into a food processor and blend for 30-second intervals until it all sticks together and is broken up.
2. Put all of the frosting ingredients into a small jug blender and blend for 1-2 minutes until smooth. Add more orange juice if there isn't liquid enough to blend.
3. Push the brownie into a pan about 8" square using your fingers.
4. Spread on the frosting then chill in the fridge for an hour to set.
5. Grate on the zest from two oranges and enjoy within 3-5 days.

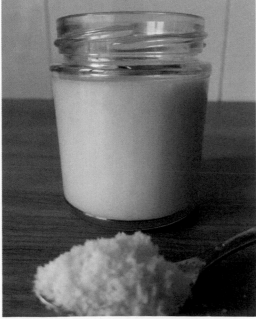

Coconut Butter

I make my own coconut butter by blending desiccated coconut into a liquid. You can do this in a powerful blender but it takes 10-15 minutes until it becomes pourable creamy butter. Make a batch of coconut butter and it will last for months in the fridge. It will be a liquid once you have blended but will become solid like coconut oil after a few hours. Made from pure coconut with nothing added.

The advantage with coconut butter is it retains the fibre and isn't just the fat extracted. Its not as smooth as coconut oil but can be used in the exact same way - melted over a double boiler then used in recipes.

A great alternative to coconut oil.

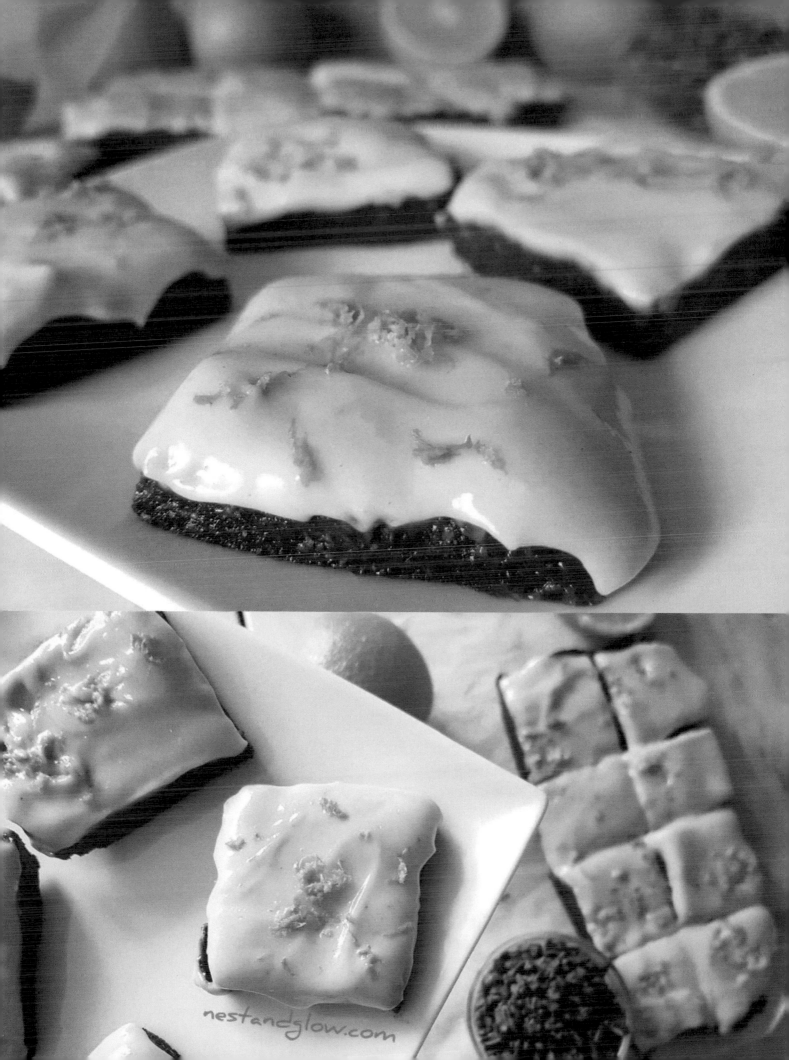

nestandglow.com

Kidney Bean and Coconut Chocolate Cake

8 Servings | 1h 20 mins **nf**

You wouldn't guess the kidney beans from the taste as even people that don't like beans or coconut have loved this cake. It's rich, chocolatey, moist and creamy despite being vegan and grain-free.

Ingredients

- 1 can **Kidney beans**, 15oz / 400ml
- 5 tbsp **Chia seeds** soaked in 15 tbsp **Water**
- 1½ cups / 150g **Desiccated coconut**
- ¾ cup / 75g **Cocoa / cacao powder**
- 1 cup / 175g pitted **Dates**
- 5 tbsp **Coconut sugar**
- 1 tsp **Vanilla**
- 1 tsp **Baking powder**
- Pinch of **Salt**
- 1 can **Coconut milk**, 14oz / 400ml
- 2 tbsp **Cacao nibs**

Equipment

- Food processor
- Electric whisk
- Oven
- Cake pan

Method

1. Preheat oven to 350F / 180C.
2. Grind chia seeds in food processor / coffee grinder until broken then soak in the water.
3. Place desiccated coconut into your food processor and blend until it starts to clump together, about a minute.
4. Add everything else to the food processor (bar the coconut milk and nibs) and blend for a few minutes until combined.
5. Spread the mixture into a lined pan about 7" in diameter.
6. Bake for about 30-35 minutes until a knife comes out clean.
7. Leave to cool and firm up – as it's gluten-free it won't become firm until cool.
8. Open your coconut milk and take off just the solid cream and leave the liquid for smoothies. Chill your can overnight if it is not separated into water and cream.
9. Whisk the coconut cream for a minute.
10. Slice the cake in half horizontally.
11. Spread the whipped coconut cream into the middle and top of the cake.

Notes

- Eat within 3 days and store in the fridge.
- Use unsweetened desiccated / shredded coconut.
- The kidney beans can be replaced by black beans if you prefer.
- If you're a coffee lover then try adding a shot of espresso to the mix.

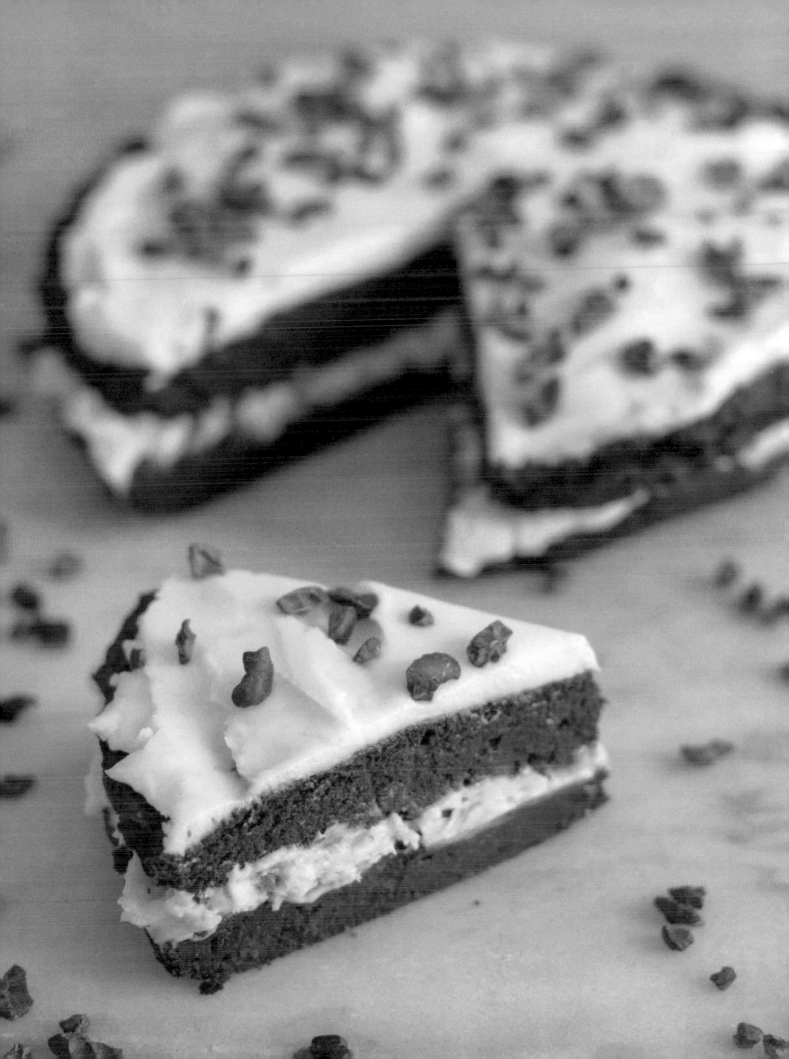

Lemon Drizzle Seed Cake

Makes 12 slices | 10 mins (raw) (p) (nf)

This raw cake is deliciously lemony and moist. Topped with a lemon coconut icing and sweetened purely with fruit. You can add a sweetener to the icing if you prefer, but I like a slightly sour lemon icing that cuts through the intense sweetness of the dried fruit.

Ingredients

- 1 cup / 175g pitted **Dates**
- 1 cup / 150g **Raisins**
- 2 cups / 280g **Sunflower seeds**
- 4 **Lemons**
- ¾ cup / 75g desiccated **Coconut**
- splash of **Water**, for blending

Equipment

- Food processor / Small blender
- 8" Square dish

Method

1. Into a food processor add the dates, raisins, sunflower seeds and the juice of two lemons.
2. Blend until the dough starts to form one big ball.
3. Spread this mixture flat into a dish.
4. Place the coconut and juice of the last two lemons into a small blender with a splash of water and blend until creamy. Add just enough water to make a creamy icing that can be spread.
5. Spread the icing on the base and sprinkle with grated lemon zest from 2 lemons.
6. Enjoy straight away or place in the fridge to firm up and eat within 5 days.

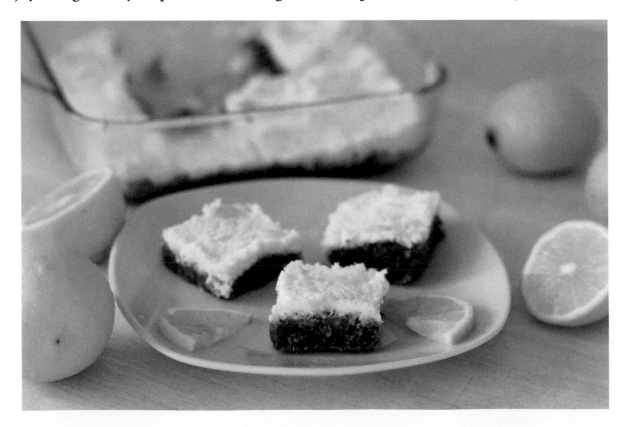

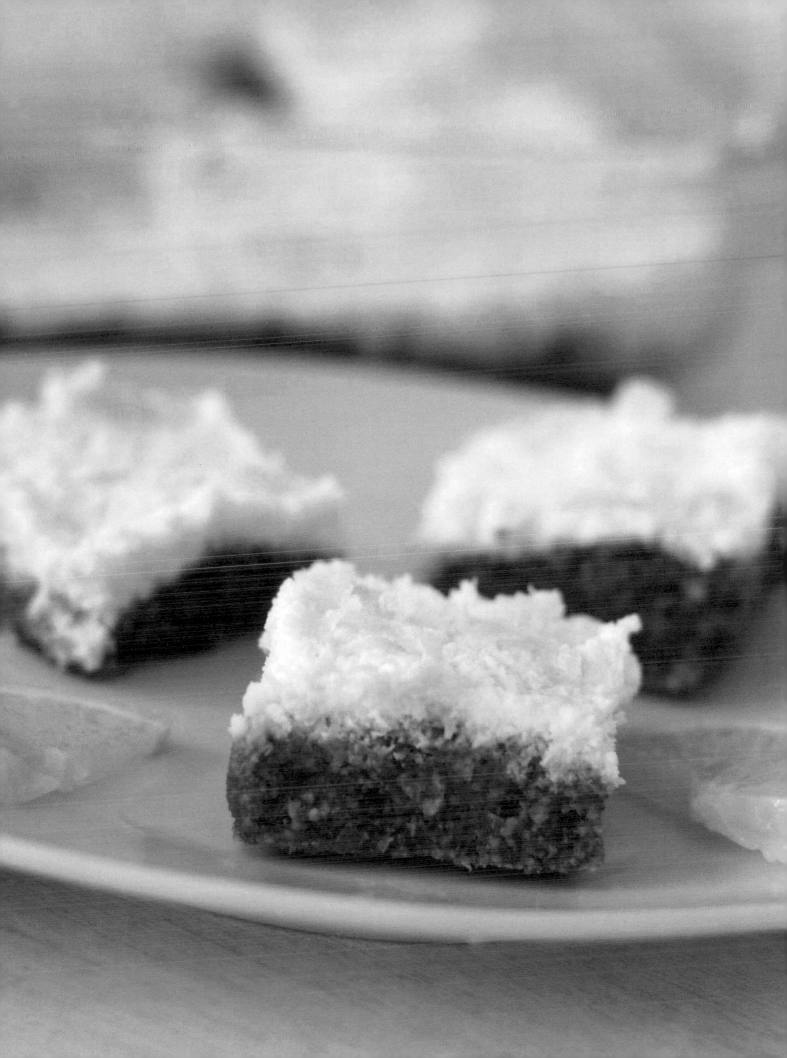

Strawberry Cheesecake Pots

Makes 4 pots | 25 mins (raw) (p)

The topping is made of strawberries sweetened with dates and thickened with chia seeds. Cashews, lemon, vanilla and a small amount of maple syrup make a zesty creamy and dreamy centre. It's bottomed off with dates, almonds and coconut all smooshed together.

Base
- 1 cup / 175g **Dates**
- 1 cup / 150g **Almonds**
- 3 tbsp **Desiccated coconut**

Cream cheese filling
- 1 cup / 150g **Cashews**
- 2 **Lemons** juiced
- 2 tbsp **Coconut oil** or **butter**, optional
- 2 tbsp **Maple syrup**
- 1 tsp **Vanilla**
- 1 cup / 240ml **Water**

Strawberry chia coulis topping
- 1 cup / 200g **Strawberries**
- ½ cup / 90g **Dates**
- 1 tbsp **Chia seeds**

Equipment
- Blender
- Jars or Tin

Method
1. Blend together all of the base ingredients until they are combined and stick together.
2. Spread out the base into your individual jars or one big pan.
3. Melt the coconut oil / butter and blend with all the other filling ingredients until smooth.
4. Pour the filling over the bases and tilt to spread to the edges.
5. Blend together the strawberry topping ingredients until the strawberries are all broken up.
6. Pour the topping over the cheesecakes.
7. Garnish with berries or mint leaves and place in the fridge for 30 minutes to set.
8. Store in the fridge and eat within a couple of days.

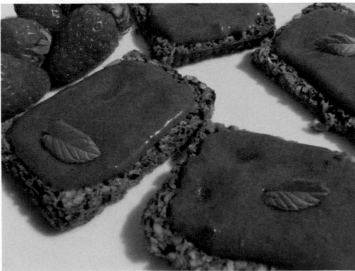

Raw Chia Jam
You can make chia jam by blending together about 1-2 cups of fresh fruit with 1 heaped tbsp of chia seeds, half of a lemon and a few dates.

This 'Jam' hasn't had any of its goodness boiled out and is perfect in place of normal jam or used in desserts. Chia seeds help to up the protein content, add heart healthy fats and naturally thicken. Keep chilled and enjoy within 3 days.

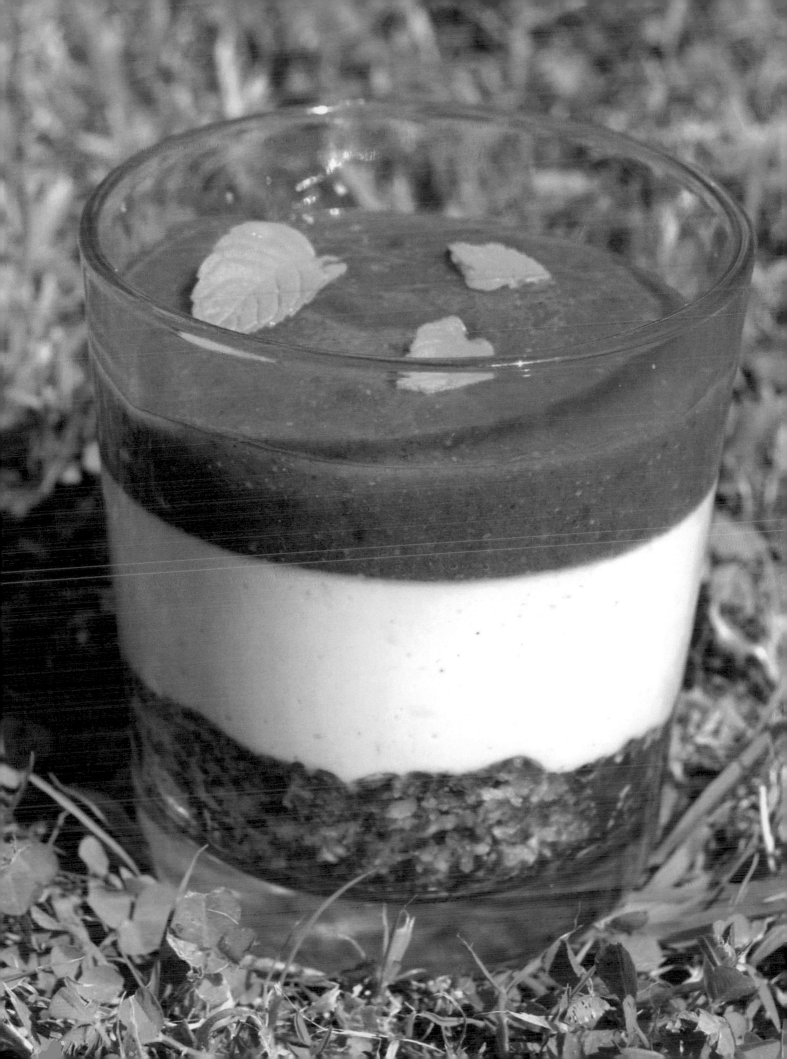

Raw Carrot Beetroot Cake with Cashew Frosting

Makes 16 servings | 25 mins 🔘raw 🔘p

This is a variation on my Carrot cake truffles but this time I've made it into one cake and suitable for grain-free and paleo diets. What can be better than a great tasting cake that makes you feel good after a slice?

Carrot Beetroot Base

- 3 cups / 450g **Carrot**, grated
- 1 large **Beetroot**, grated
- 1 cup / 150g **Walnuts**
- 1 cup / 175g **Dates**
- ½ cup / 75g **Raisins**
- 1 cup / 100g shredded **Coconut**
- 1 tsp **Cinnamon**
- 1 tsp ground **Ginger**
- ½ tsp **Nutmeg**
- a pinch of **Salt**

Cashew Vanilla Icing

- ¾ cup / 115g **Cashew nuts**
- 2-4 tbsp **Sweetener** such as Maple syrup
- 1 tsp **Vanilla**
- 2 tbsp **Coconut butter** or **oil**, optional
- a splash of **Water** for blending

Equipment

- Blender
- Tin 8" square

Method

1. Place everything for the base (except the carrot and beetroot) and blend until they start to break down.
2. Separate the base mixture into two.
3. Blend half of the mixture with 2/3 of the carrots until combined.
4. Blend the other half with the rest of carrots and all the beetroot.
5. Melt the coconut oil / butter and blend all of the frosting ingredients together until smooth.
6. Layer on the bases in the tin and then pour and spread the frosting on top.
7. Place in the fridge to set for at least an hour and enjoy within 3 days.

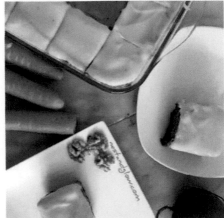

Juice Pulp Cakes

This recipe is similar to the cakes I make from the pulp left over when juicing.

After juicing sweet fruit or vegetables you can whizz the pulp with spices, dried fruit and nuts to make a cake. Press into a tin and top with any of the many frostings / icings listed in this book.

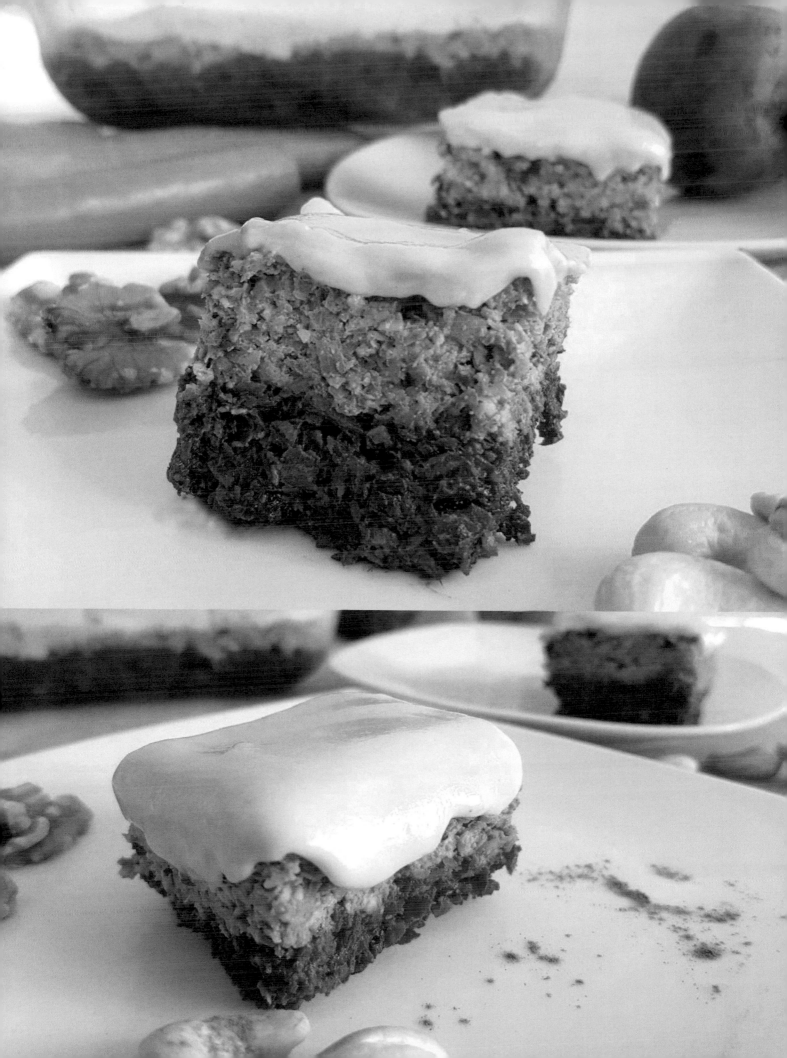

Tropical Lemon Cake

Yields **12 servings** | **45** mins

Pineapple and coconut base with tangy mango lemon frosting. This tropical lemon cake is perfect for a summer's day. It's no bake, so easy and quick to make - just blend the base and topping, then layer in a tin.

Base

- 1 medium **Pineapple**, cubed, skinned and core removed
- ⅔ cup / 100g **Raisins**
- 1 cup / 150g **Buckwheat**
- 1 cup / 140g **Sunflower seeds**
- 1 cup / 100g **Desiccated coconut**
- 2 **Carrots**, grated

Topping

- 2 **Lemons**, juiced
- 1 cup / 150g **Cashews**
- 1 **Mango**, cubed
- 4 tbsp **Maple syrup**
- 4 tablespoons **Coconut butter / oil**
- **Turmeric**, just a pinch to add colour

Equipment

- Blender
- Cake tin 8"square or Jars

Method

1. Blend together all of the base ingredients until they are combined and stick together.
2. Spread out the base into your individual jars or one big pan.
3. Melt the coconut oil / butter and then blend with all the other filling ingredients until smooth.
4. Pour the filling over the bases and tilt to spread to the edges.
5. Garnish with coconut and place in the fridge for 30 minutes to set.
6. Store in the fridge and eat within a couple of days.

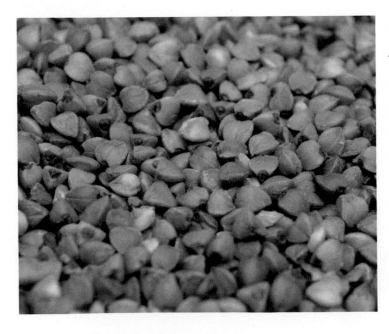

Buckwheat

This rather confusingly named seed is not related to wheat and is suitable for grain and gluten free diets. It's known as a pseudograin as its often used like a grain.

Buckwheat is inexpensive and can be sprouted to make it more digestible. It's one of my most used staple ingredients. Useful in cakes, porridge, risottos and waffles to name a few.

One of my most common breakfasts is **buckwheat** spouted overnight then rinsed and eaten with **apple**, **raisins** and **cinnamon**.

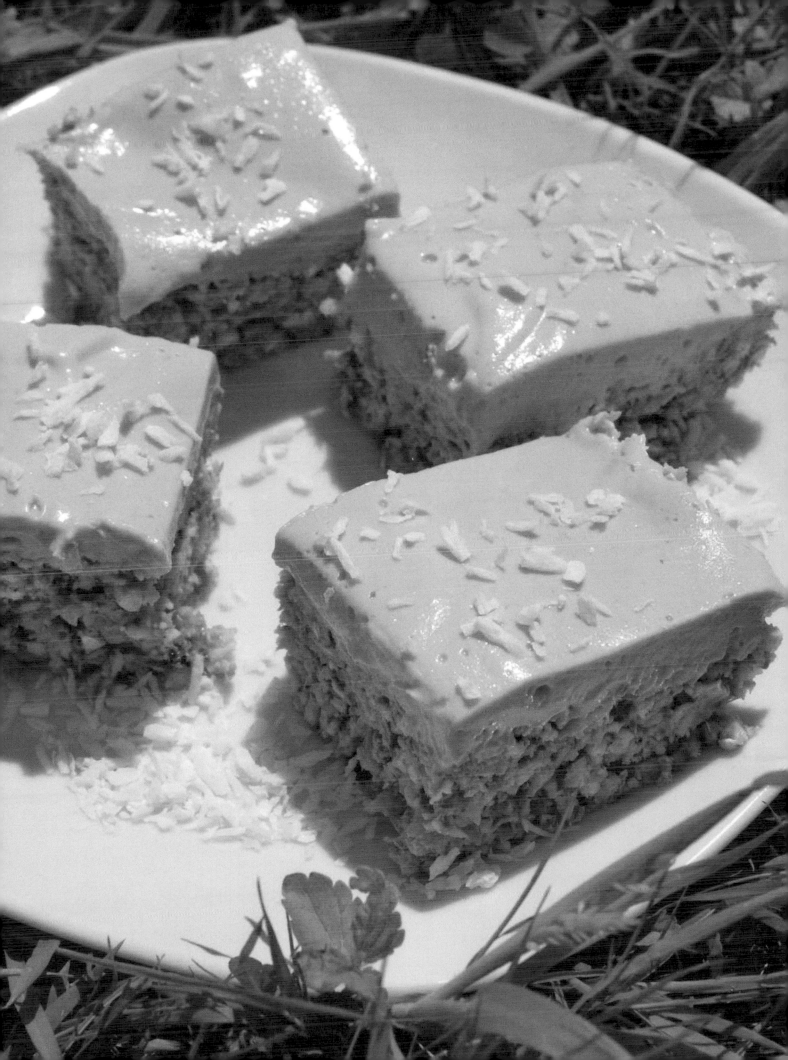

Mocha Chocolate Cashew Cheesecake

Makes 10 slices| 25 mins (raw) (p)

Cream cheese and eggs have been ditched in favour of heart-healthy cashew nuts and coconut butter. I would also consider this cake suitable for a raw vegan diet – but you will probably want to use a coffee substitute such as chicory.

Base

- 1 cup / 140g **Almonds**
- 1 cup / 175g pitted **Dates**
- ½ cup / 30g shredded **Coconut**
- 2 tbsp **Cacao powder**
- a pinch of **Salt**

Topping suggestions

- **Cacao nibs** or **Coffee beans**

Equipment

- Blender / food processor
- Spring form 8" tin and Bain-marie

Filling

- 1½ cups / 225g **Cashews**
- 3.5 oz / 100g **Coconut Butter** (page 10)
- 1 shot **Espresso** or **Chicory coffee**
- 5 tbsp **Coconut Sugar** (page 90)
- 2 tbsp **Cacao powder**
- 1 tsp **Vanilla**
- 1 tsp **Cinnamon**
- 1 cup / 235ml **Water** (add more if needed)

Method

1. Blend all of the base ingredients in a food processor until they stick together and the oils from the almonds start to be released.
2. Push the base into a cake tin about 8" in diameter.
3. Melt the coconut butter in a bain-marie.
4. Add all of the filling ingredients to a high-speed blender and blend on high for 2-3 minutes until smooth.
5. Pour the filling over the base and chill in the fridge for a few hours or one hour in the freezer.
6. Sprinkle on the cacao / coffee beans, store in the fridge and enjoy within 3 days.

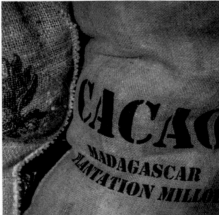

Cacao and Cocoa

These sound similar and can be used interchangeably but are different products:

Cacao is the purest form of chocolate and it is usually raw and minimally processed. It's thought to be the food highest in antioxidants. In this book I use cacao nibs, powder and butter.

Cocoa has been heat treated and more refined, but is still a very nutritious ingredient as long as it's pure without sugar added.

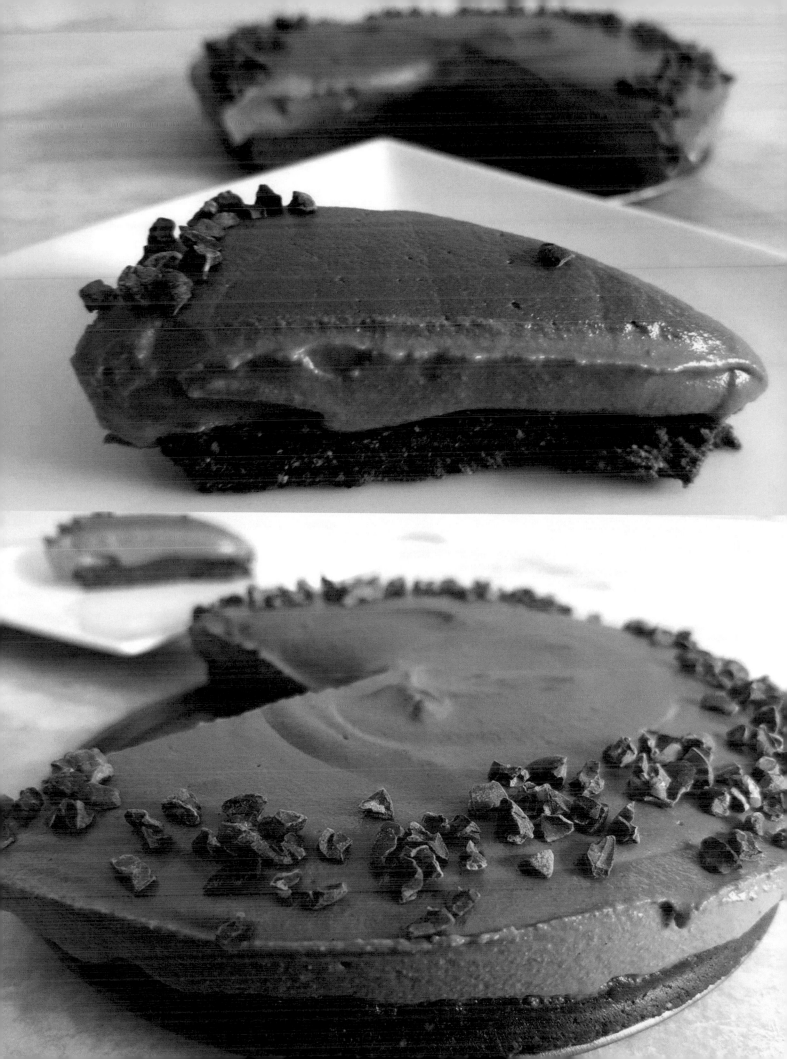

Raw Pumpkin Pie Cake

Makes 16 servings | 25 mins (raw) (p)

It's easily one of my favourite raw cakes these days and like all Nest and Glow recipes is super easy – just blend and chill. If you want to eat it as a pie simply push the base into a pie case (individual or one big one).

Topping

- 1 cup / 150g, **Cashews**
- 2-4 tbsp **Coconut sugar** – or any other sweetener like maple / date syrup
- 2 tbsp **Coconut butter** or **oil**
- 4 tbsp **Pumpkin / butternut squash**, grated
- 1 tsp **Ginger**, diced
- 1 tsp **Cinnamon**
- 1 tsp **Turmeric**
- 1 tsb **Vanilla extract** or half a bean
- **Water**, just enough to blend

Base

- 1 cup / 150g **Walnuts**
- 1 cup / 175g **Dates**
- 3 tbsp **Coconut**, desiccated

Equipment

- Food processor / blender
- Cake tin or pie case

Method

1. Pulse together all of the base ingredients until they are all broken up and stick together.
2. Either push the base into a dish or pie case.
3. Put the base in the fridge while you make the topping.
4. Add all topping ingredients together and then whizz until smooth.
5. You will need to add some water (about 3-4 tbsp) so that the blender can whizz the topping.
6. Pour the topping on, chill for an hour and it's ready to eat. Consume within a few days.
7. You can put this cake / pie in the freezer and take out an hour before to defrost and it will last months. I like to slice up before freezing and defrost a slice at a time.

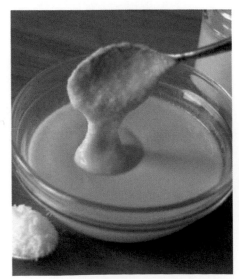

Oil Free Adaptations

I use extra virgin olive oil and cold-pressed raw virgin coconut oil in some recipes. The olive oil can just be left out or replaced with water.

Raw virgin coconut oil is used in some desserts to help them set. If you are avoiding oil then you can replace this with a 100% pure no added oil nut or seed butter. You can make these yourself, see Coconut Butter (page 10) or Sprouted Almond Butter (page 76). These will need warming like coconut oil to become runny. Coconut (shown left), sunflower and almond butter all work well to replace oil.

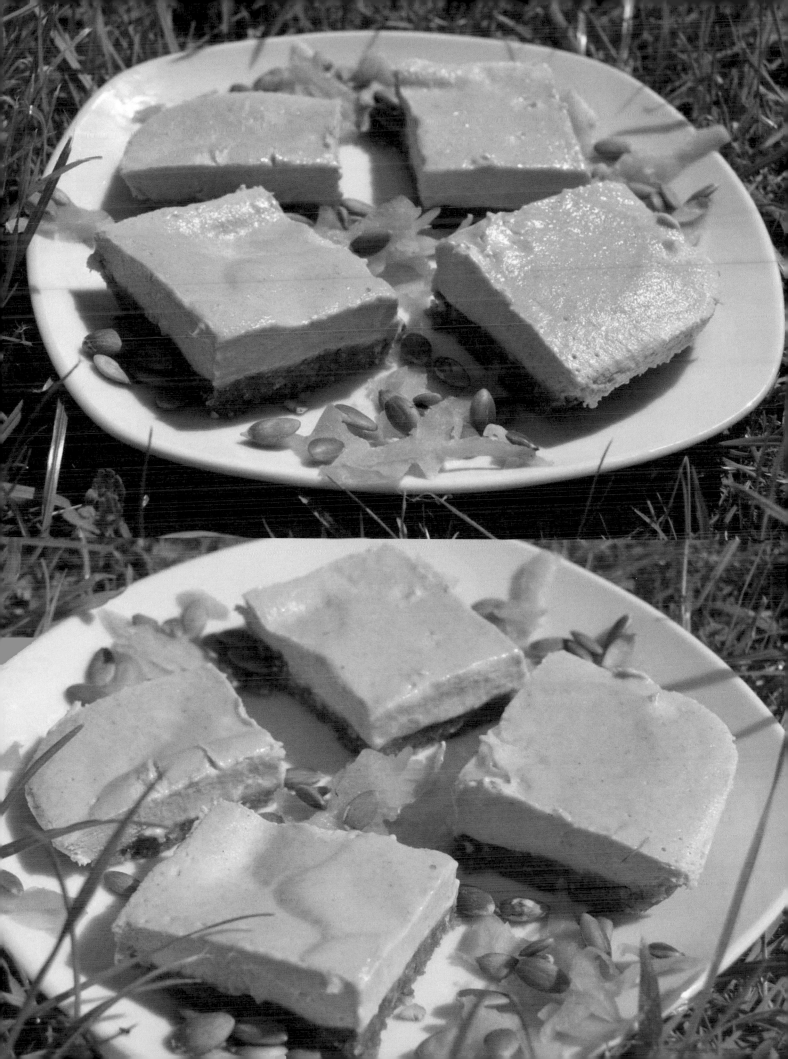

Raw Chocolate Cashew Thumbprints

Makes 12 thumbprints | 20 mins **raw** **p**

Raw Chocolate thumbprint filled with cashew vanilla cream. These sweets have a fudgy and chewy texture. You can use any other nut in place of the almonds.

Ingredients

- 1¼ cups / 200g **Almonds**
- 1½ cups / 220g **Raisins**
- 3 tbsp **Cacao powder**
- pinch of **Salt**
- ½ cup / 75g **Cashews**
- 1 tsp **Vanilla extract**
- 2 tbsp **Maple syrup**
- 2 tbsp **Coconut oil or butter**, melted
- **Water**, for blending

Equipment

- Food processor / small blender

Method

1. Place the almonds, raisins, cacao and salt into a food processor and blend until it all sticks together (1-2 minutes).
2. Roll the raw chocolate dough into balls and then press with your thumb to leave an imprint.
3. Blend all the remaining ingredients for the icing in a small blender with just enough water to blend smooth.
4. Fill the thumbprints with the icing and enjoy as they are or chill to firm up.
5. Store in the fridge and eat within about 3 days.

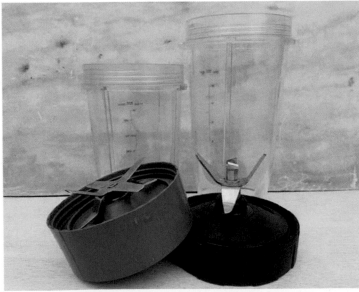

Blender

The most common question I get asked is what blender do I use and what do I recommend.

95% of the time I use a small jug / bullet blender where the blade screws onto the bottom. Just make sure to get one that is at least 600w and you will be able to make everything in this book. Sometimes the small size means you will need to do it in batches, shaking or scraping down the sides but it will still get the job done.

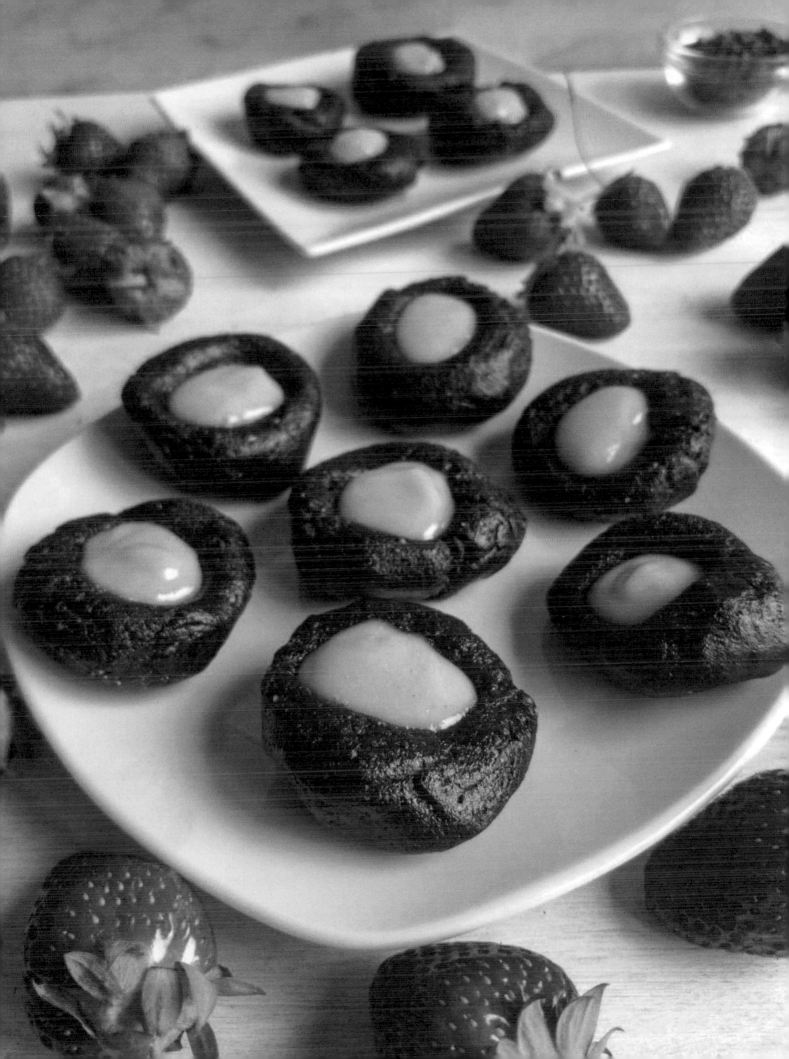

Fruit Juice Jelly Sweets

Makes 24-48 sweets depending on mould size | 20 mins **p** **nf**

These fruit juice jelly sweets are made of just 3 ingredients; fruit juice, the seaweed agar agar and a sweetener. They are quick and easy to make. Agar agar is a really fun ingredient to play with as it sets liquids and can be used to make many things like cheeses and sweets.

Ingredients

- 250ml / 1 cup **Juice**
- 1 tbsp **Agar Agar Powder** (page 94)
- 2 tbsp **Maple syrup** / xylitol / sweetener

Equipment

- Blender and sieve or Juicer
- Pan
- Silicon moulds

Fruit and juice

Use pre-made or juice fresh fruit

- **Orange**
- **Pineapple**
- **Plums**
- **Kiwi** (I didn't wash out between boiling the plum and ended up with black)
- **Apple**

Method

1. Place the mould in the freezer.
2. Stir the agar agar and sweetener into the juice until dissolved.
3. Bring to the boil. Simmer for 5 minutes stirring constantly while making a figure of 8 and 0.
4. Take off the heat and let cool for 2 minutes.
5. Pour into the moulds and place in the freezer. Don't worry if the mixture spills over the mould, this excess can just be pulled off when it is out of the mould.
6. Take out of the freezer after 5 minutes and pop out of the moulds.
7. As they are fresh they wont last like normal jelly sweets. Store in the fridge and enjoy a few days after making, mine often don't last an hour.

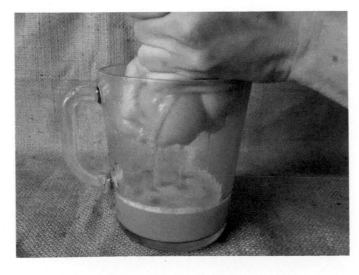

Blender Juicing

These jelly sweets can be made by using up fruit past its best.

If you don't have a juicer you can just use a blender to liquidise. Then strain off the pulp by either squeezing in a Nut Milk Bag (page 124) or by using a sieve and a pushing with a spoon.

You may need to add a dash of water to help the blender whiz up the fruit.

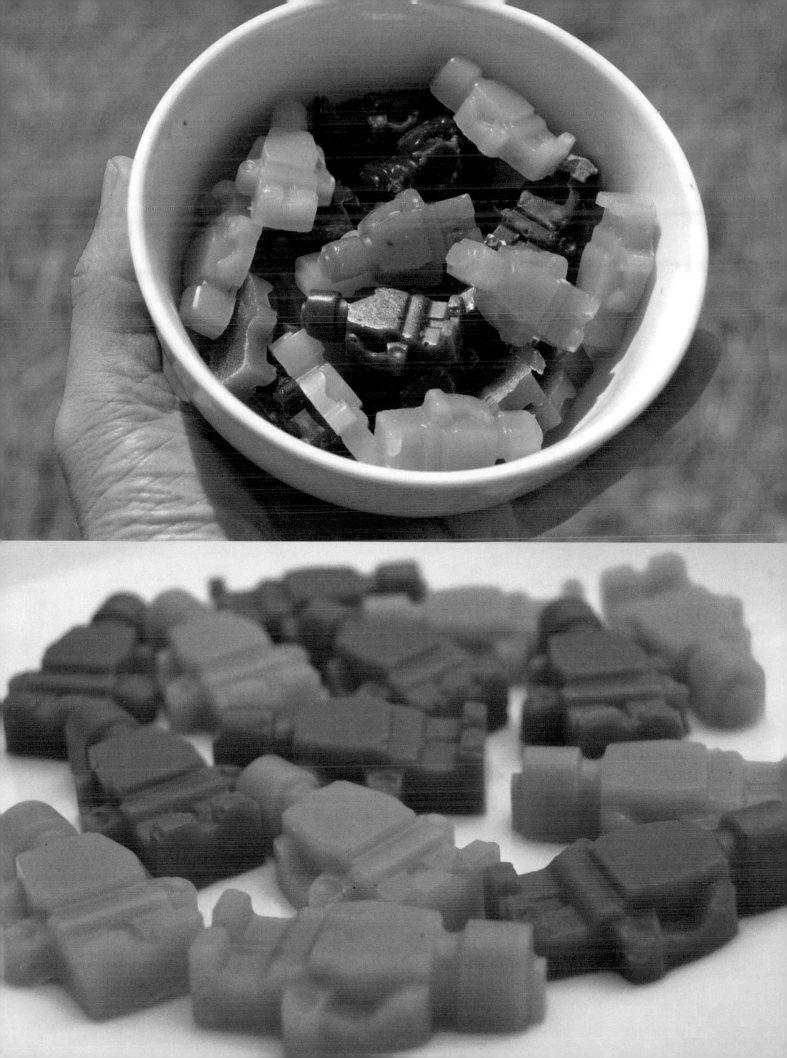

Almond Stuffed Raw Chocolate Covered Dates

Makes 5 sweets | 20 mins **raw** **p**

These little delicious indulgent chocolate covered stuffed dates are easy and fun to make. Medjool dates on their own are a delicious healthy natural fudge but add a crunchy almond or two and coat in a crispy layer of rich dark chocolate for the perfect healthy chocolate sweet.

Ingredients

- 5 **Medjool dates**
- 10-15 **Almonds**
- 2 tbsp **Cacao / cocoa powder**
- 2 tbsp **Sweetener** / maple / agave / coconut nectar / any
- ⅓ cup / 80 ml **Coconut oil or butter**
- 3 crushed **Almonds** to top

Equipment

- Double boiler / bain-marie
- Greaseproof paper

Method

1. Carefully open the Medjool date lengthways and remove the stone and stem. Try to split the date down the middle, but it doesn't matter too much if you mess this up as the soft date is very malleable.
2. Insert an almond or three depending on the size of the dates / almonds then fold the date back and squeeze shut.
3. Place in the freezer for 5 minutes while you make the chocolate coating.
4. Melt the coconut oil / butter and then mix with the cacao and sweetener until smooth.
5. Coat all the dates with the chocolate. Either dip and roll in the chocolate or spoon over the chocolate while holding on a fork. Place on greaseproof paper and freeze for 5 minutes.

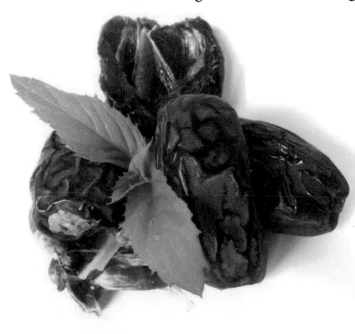

Medjool Dates

These are a variety of dates known for being rich, soft and chewy with an almost caramel like taste. They are nature's own fudge.

There are hundreds of other varieties of dates but medjool are often known as 'the King of dates.' They are labour intensive to produce so are often the most expensive.

You can use any variety of date interchangeably when they are blended but for this sweet I do recommend medjools. Normal dates (often deglet noor) can be soaked in water to become softer, easier to blend and more similar to Medjool Dates.

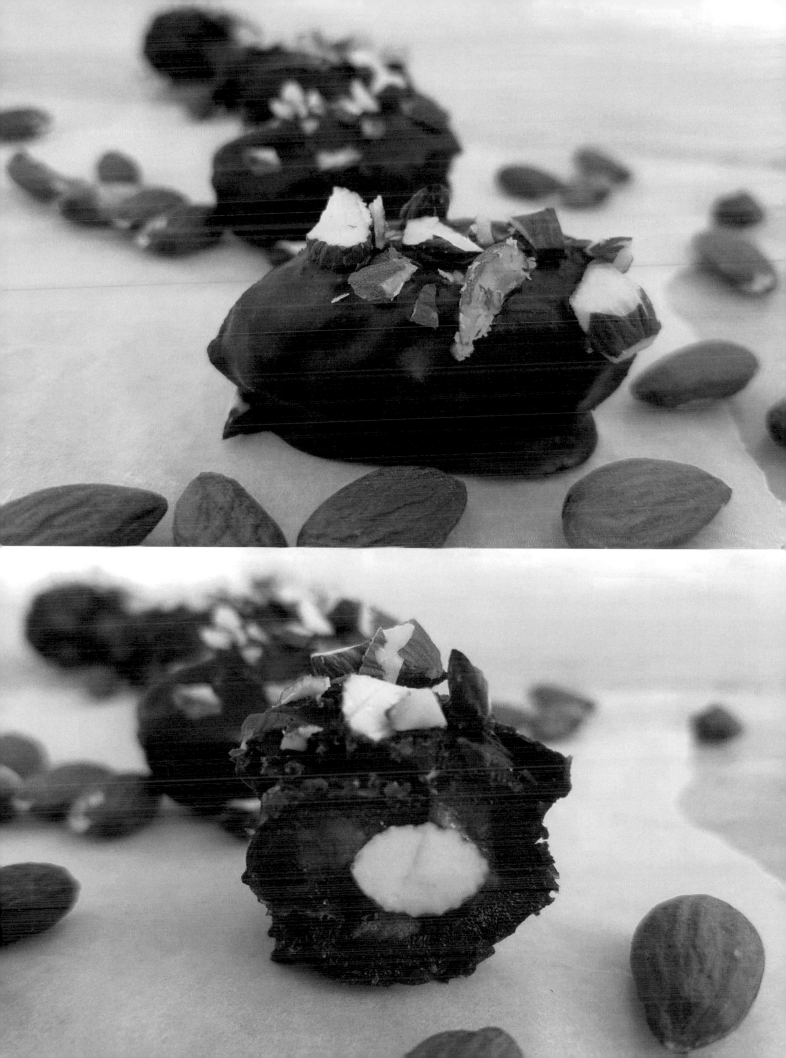

Peanut Chocolate Ice Cream Bars

Makes 6 bars| 3h 15 mins

These are a much healthier version of the popular peanut chocolate bars. They are full of pure ingredients and contain many vitamins and minerals.

The bars may take a few hours to make, but most of this time is the freezer doing the work. The high-fat content of the coconut milk and the cashew nuts mixed with the aeration of blending them means that no churning is needed and they are soft like an ice cream bar.

Ingredients

- 1 cup / 150g soaked **Cashew nuts**
- 1 cup / 240ml **Coconut milk,** full fat
- 6 tbsp **Maple syrup**
- 1 tsp **Vanilla extract**
- 4 tbsp **Almond / Peanut butter**, chunky
- 5.3oz / 150g **Chocolate,**your favourite type
- 1 tbsp chopped **Nuts** (any such as almonds, peanuts, hazelnuts)

Equipment

- Blender
- Double boiler
- 6" approx square dish
- Greaseproof / parchment paper

Method

1. Mix together 2 tbsp of maple syrup with the nut butter and spread into the dish. It's best to use a flexible pan or a normal pan with a non-stick paper to make it easy to take out.
2. If you are using tinned coconut milk shake it up and mix so all the coconut cream is evenly distributed.
3. Add the cashews, coconut milk, 4 tbsp of maple syrup and the vanilla to a high-speed blender and whizz until all is combined. You may need to add a few tbsp of water to help the blender make it smooth.
4. Pour over the vanilla ice cream mixture over the nut butter in the dish.
5. Place this in the freezer for about 3 hours. Remove when it's frozen but still soft enough to slide a knife in.
6. Tip out of the dish and it should be soft enough to cut, but hard enough to work with.
7. Cut in half, then cut each of these into three so you have 6 ice cream bars.
8. Chop up the chocolate and melt using a double boiler.
9. Using a fork hold each bar over the melted chocolate and spoon on enough chocolate to cover.
10. Sprinkle with the chopped nuts, place on non stick paper and freeze for half an hour.
11. They will be ready to eat or you can store in the freezer for a few months.
12. Take out of the freezer for 30 minutes, if frozen for more than 4 hours to soften before eating.

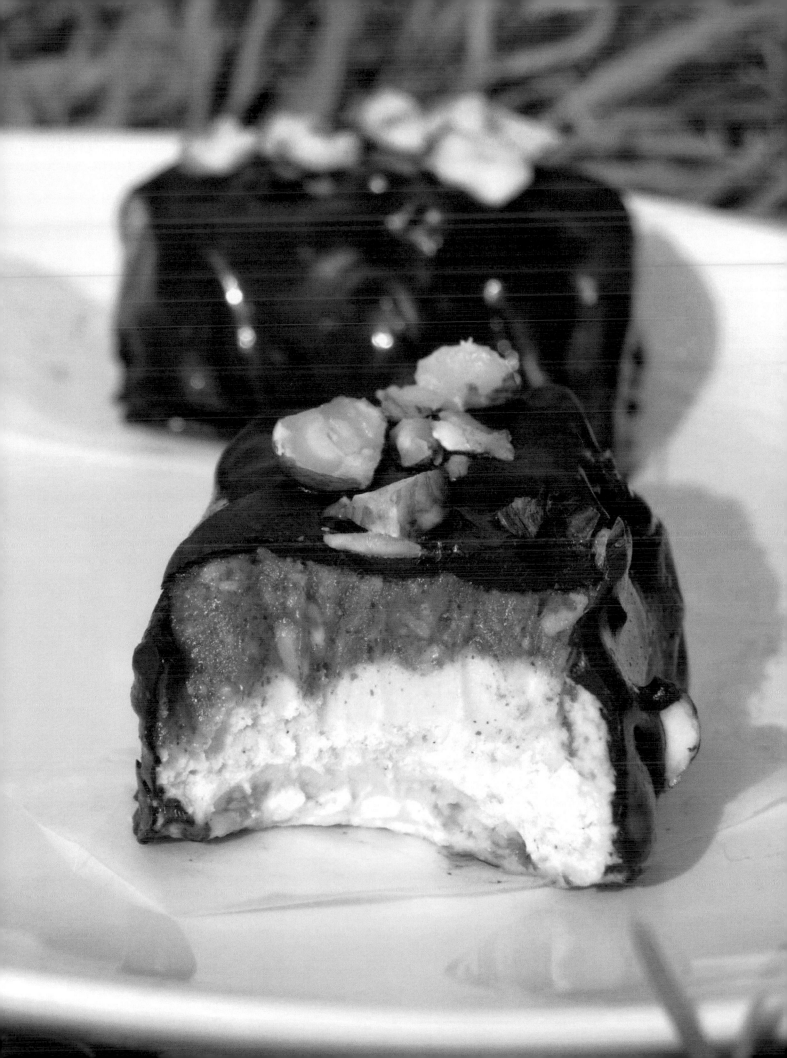

Chocolate Hazelnut Fudge

Makes 16 fudge squares | 30 mins (raw) (p)

This Chocolate Hazelnut Fudge has the taste of chocolate spread like nutella but is made from pure natural ingredients. The creaminess of the cashews help to give a milk chocolate taste to this dairy free recipe. Also the cashews add sweetness and reduce the amount of sweetener needed.

Ingredients

- 1 cup / 150g **Cashew nuts**
- 1 cup / 150g **Hazelnuts** + 1 tbsp chopped for decoration
- 4 tbsp **Cacao / Cocoa powder**
- 1 tsp **Vanilla extract**
- 4-6 tbsp **Maple / Date syrup** / sweetener
- ½ cup / 120ml **Coconut oil** or **Butter**

Equipment

- Small blender / Coffee grinder
- Double boiler / Bain-marie
- Dish 6" square

Method

1. Using a double boiler / bain-marie melt the coconut oil / butter.
2. Grind the cashew and hazelnuts into a fine powder using a coffee grinder or blender with a small jug. They should just be starting to stick and release their oils.
3. Mix together the ground nuts, cocoa powder, vanilla, melted coconut and sweetener. I usually use 4 tbsp of maple syrup, but you might like to add more if you want a sweeter fudge.
4. Pour this mixture out into a square dish about 6". Spread out and smooth the top with a spatula. No need to grease as the fudge has enough natural fats.
5. Sprinkle with 1 tbsp of chopped hazelnuts and push these into the fudge.
6. Place in the fridge for 30 minutes to set.
7. Remove from the fridge and run a knife around the outside. Then you should be able to pull the fudge out and put on to a flat surface.
8. Cut into 16 squares and enjoy immediately. Stored in the fridge it will last for several weeks.

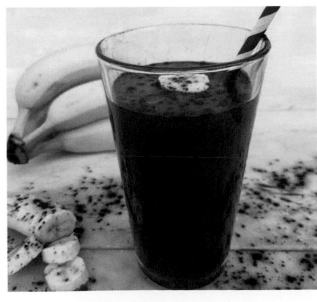

Banana Fudge Milkshake

- 2 **Bananas**, frozen work best
- ¼ cup / 35 g **Hazelnuts**
- 1-2 tbsp **Cocoa / Cacao**
- 6 **Dates**, pitted
- 1 cup / 250 ml **Water**

Blend together everything and enjoy this milkshake that serves two!

It's recommended to use frozen bananas or chilled water to make the drink chilled.

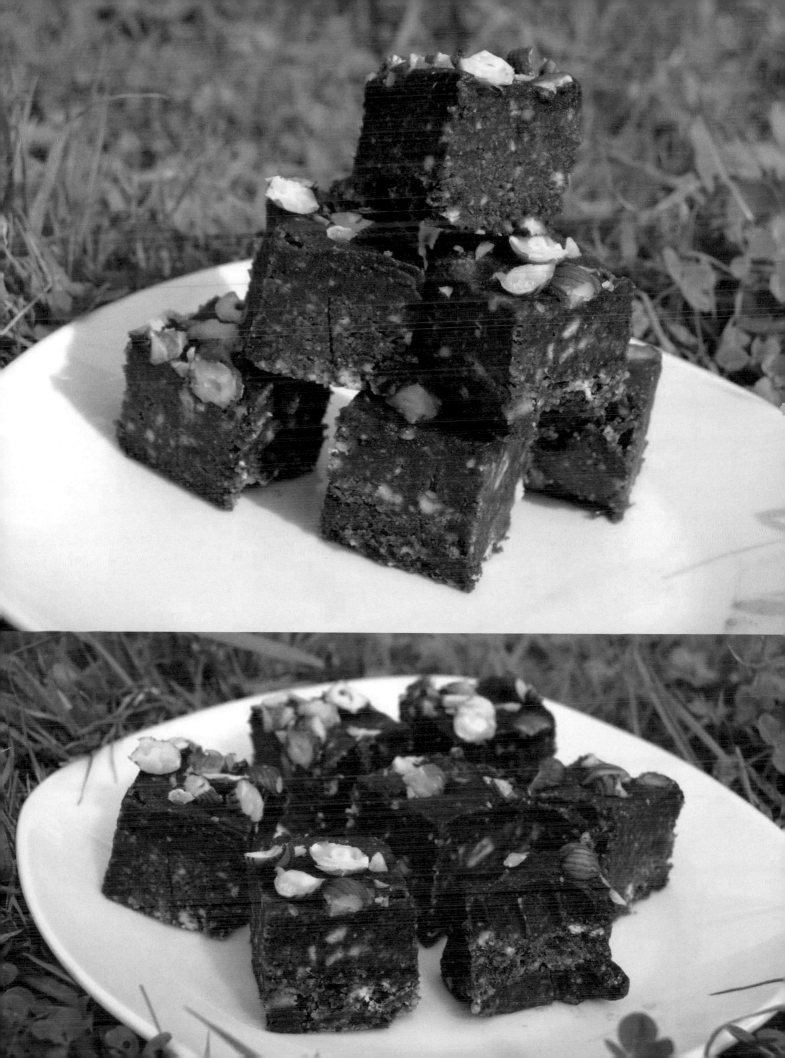

Sunflower Caramel Dark Chocolate Cups

Makes 24 cups | 10 mins

Homemade sunflower seed caramel is surrounded by dark bitter chocolate in these easy to make sweets. Sunflower seed caramel cups taste similar to traditional peanut butter cups but are free of dairy, nuts, refined sugar and palm oil.

Ingredients

- 8.8oz / 250g **Dark chocolate**
- 2 cups / 280g **Sunflower seeds**
- 4-8 tbsp **Maple syrup**, coconut nectar or similar sweetener
- 1 tbsp **Molasses**
- 1 tsp **Vanilla**
- a pinch of **Salt**

Equipment

- Food processor / small blender
- Small silicone cup cases
- Oven
- Double boiler

Raw version (raw)

- To make this raw, sprout and dehydrate the seeds rather than baking.

Method

1. Spread the sunflower seeds on a pan and roast for 10-12 minutes at 375F/ 190C.
2. Take out of the oven as soon as a few turn golden. Watch like a hawk as they can burn quickly.
3. Leave to cool for 10 minutes.
4. Place the warm seeds along with everything else apart from the chocolate into a blender and pulse blend to make a paste.
5. Depending on your blender you may need to scrape down the sides and blend for several minutes until it combines.
6. Melt 3/4 of the chocolate in a double boiler then take off the heat and stir in the last 1/4 until melted. This is for easy tempering of the chocolate to give the right snap and glossy look.
7. Pour half of the chocolate into the cases and then chill for a few minutes to set.
8. Press the sunflower caramel into the cases then cover with the remaining chocolate.
9. Sprinkle with sunflower seeds and chill to set.

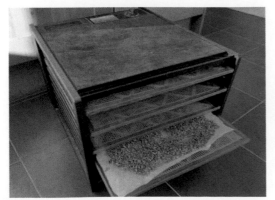

Dehydrator

This is an appliance that's designed for drying food. It's super useful in a healthy kitchen and has many uses. I use mine mainly to dry sprouted nuts / seeds and make raw food like kale crisps and crackers. It's foolproof making healthy snacks like kale crisps as it's impossible to burn them. The downside is it often takes 10-12 hours to make something. They can be picked up relatively inexpensively.

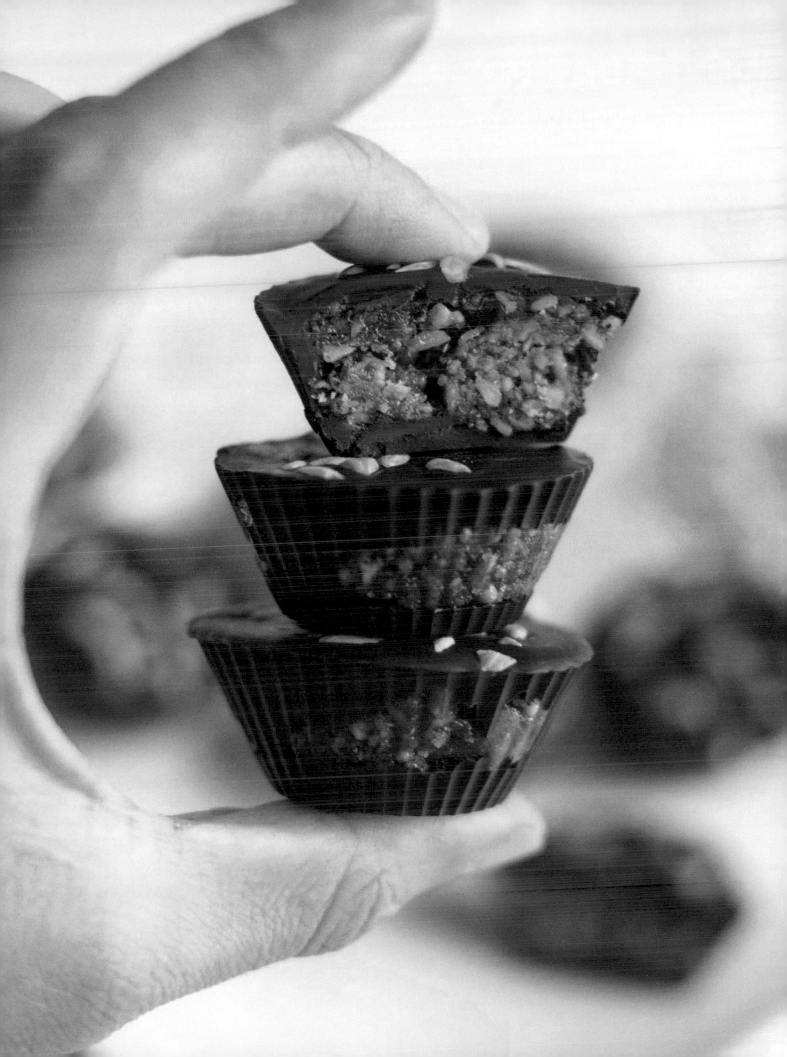

Calcium Chocolate Fudge

Makes 16 squares | 20 mins

This easy vegan fudge combines some of the highest plant based sauces of calcium such as sesame seeds, figs, almonds and molasses to make a delicious fudge.

One piece provides over 35% of your RDA of calcium for a healthy adult – about 251 mg. For children aged 1-3 one square provides 70% of their calcium RDA and for children aged 4-10 a single square provides about 50% of their RDA of calcium.

Calcium Fudge

- 2 cups / 280g **Sesame seeds**
- 1 cup / 140g **Almonds**
- 1 cup / 150g dried **Figs**, stems removed
- 1 cup **Raisins**
- 5 tbsp **Blackstrap molasses**
- 4 tbsp **Cacao/Cocoa powder**
- 1 tbsp **Cinnamon**

Chocolate Avocado Frosting

- 2 **Avocados**
- 4-6 tbsp **Sweetener** such as Maple syrup
- 2 tbsp **Coconut oil**, you can leave out if you prefer but the icing won't set as firm
- 4 tbsp **Cacao / Cocoa powder**

Equipment

- Blender and 8" Pan

Method

1. Place the sesame seeds and almonds into your food processor and blend for a few minutes until broken up.
2. Add everything else for the fudge into the food processor and blend for a few minutes until it all sticks together in a ball.
3. Turn out the fudge into a pan about 8" square and press down.
4. Blend all of the frosting ingredients together in a small jug, you may need to add a few tbsp of water.
5. Spread the icing over the fudge and chill to set. Take out of pan and slice into squares.
6. Will last for three days in the fridge with the frosting or several weeks without the frosting and can be frozen.

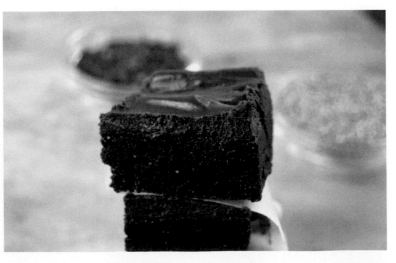

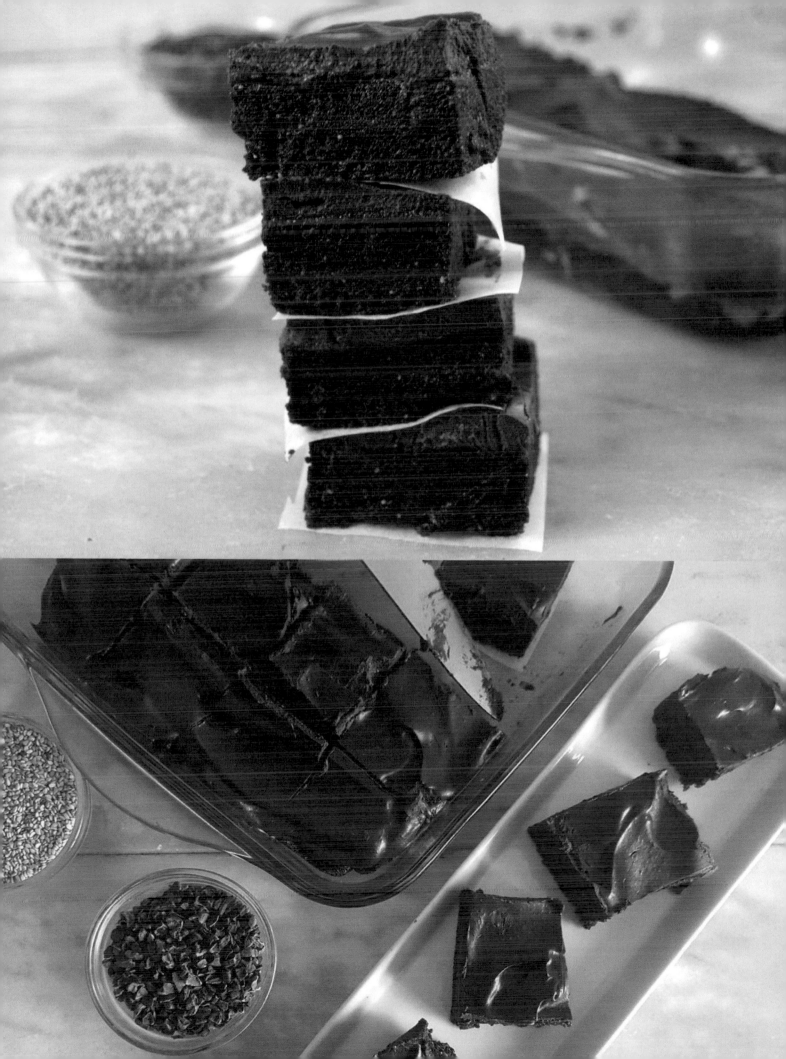

Vanilla Fudge & Natural Sprinkles

Makes 16 fudge squares | 30 mins (raw) (p)

Natural and healthy food without nasties doesn't mean a world of grey! These sprinkles are made from coconut with fruit, veg, spices and seaweed. They work really well in recipes like this raw vanilla cashew fudge.

Vanilla Fudge

- 1 cup / 150g **Cashews**
- 7oz / 200g **Coconut butter**
- 4 tbsp **Maple syrup**
- 1 tsp **Vanilla extract**
- 6 tbsp **Natural sprinkles**

Equipment

- Blender and Non-stick sheets
- Oven / dehydrator and 6" Dish

Natural Organic Sprinkles

- ¼ cup / 25g **Shredded coconut**
- 2-4 tbsp **Fruit / Veg juice:**
  - **Spirulina** or **Wheatgrass** mixed with water
  - **Carrot juice** or **Turmeric** with water
  - **Red cabbage** or **Blackberries** juiced
  - **Red cabbage** and **baking soda**
  - **Beetroot juice**

Method

1. Put the cashews in a small blender or coffee grinder and then grind until broken down into a powder.
2. Melt the coconut butter then stir into the ground cashews along with the syrup and vanilla.
3. Blend several times and stir in between until everything is combined. Don't worry if there is some liquid fat separation, this is normal.
4. Stir in 3 tbsp of natural sprinkles then spread out in a dish that's about 6" square.
5. Using a spatula smooth over the top of the fudge.
6. Sprinkle on 3 tbsp of natural sprinkles and then place in the freezer for half an hour to firm up.
7. Run a knife around the outside of the fudge to release it and then slice into squares
8. Enjoy immediately or store in the fridge and eat within a few days.

Organic sprinkles

1. Mix about 2 tablespoons of fruit / veg juice with ¼ cup / 25g of natural shredded coconut.
2. If you're using a powder such as wheat grass or turmeric mix ½ tsp with 2 tbsp of water.
3. Once the coconut is dyed, spread out over a non-stick sheet.
4. Place in an oven on a very low heat, preferably less than 100C, with the door slightly open. They should be dry in 50-60 minutes depending on the temperature, but check them every 10 minutes to make sure they don't burn. Toss while drying to speed it up.
5. If you have a food dehydrator, put them in at 100f / 40C and they should be dry in 4-6 hours.
6. Store in an airtight container somewhere dark and they will be good for a few months. However it's better to use them sooner rather than later as the colour and flavour will fade.

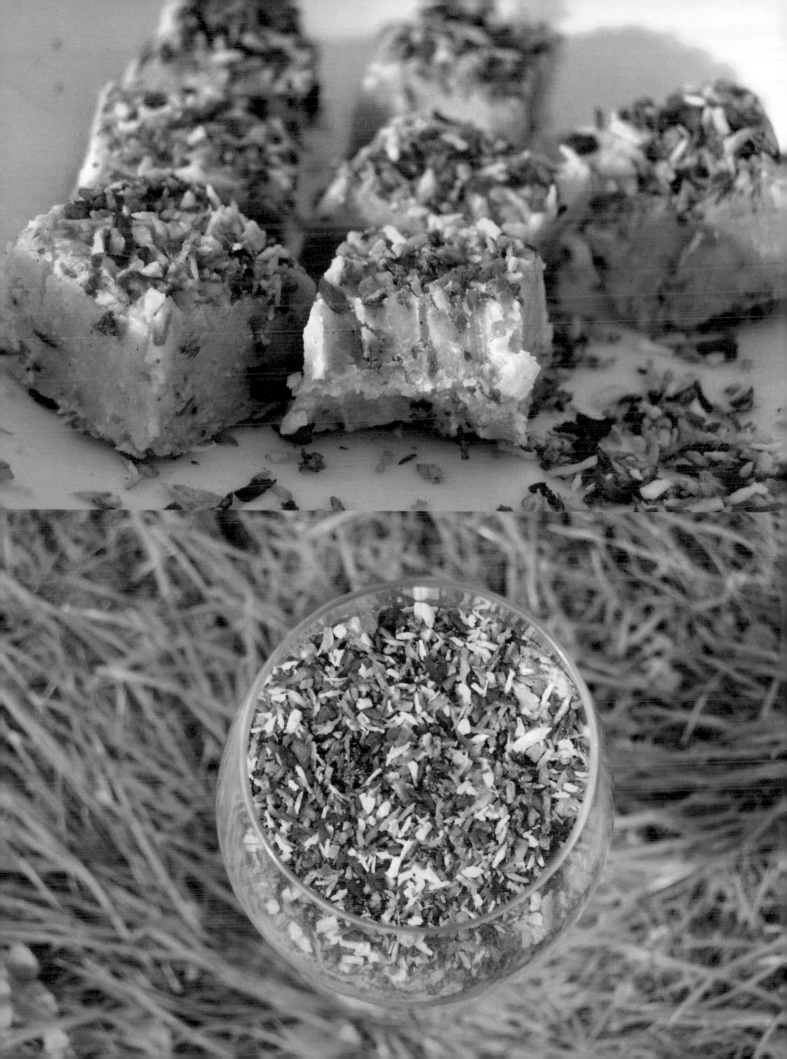

Halva Sesame Chocolate Raisin Balls

Makes 24 balls | 10mins (raw) (p) (nf)

These little chocolate sesame halva balls can be made in a few minutes and are the perfect on the go energy snack. Full of protein, heart healthy fats, calcium and fibre.

Ingredients
- 1 cup / 140g **Sesame seeds**
- 1 cup / 150g **Raisins**
- ½ cup / 50g **Cacao / Cocoa powder**

Equipment
- Food processor / small blender

Method
1. Place everything into a blender or food processor.
2. Blend until it starts to stick together.
3. You may need to scrape the sides or shake your jug a few times between blends.
4. Scoop about a heaped tea spoon and roll into firm balls.
5. Store in an air-tight container in the fridge, where they will be good for a few weeks.

Energy Balls

You can make energy balls out of any dried fruit and nut or seed. Just blend together and add flavourings such as cacao, cinnamon, cayenne pepper or wheat-grass. It's so easy to make your own energy balls. Stored somewhere air-tight in the fridge they will last for weeks and always be on hand for when you need a boost.

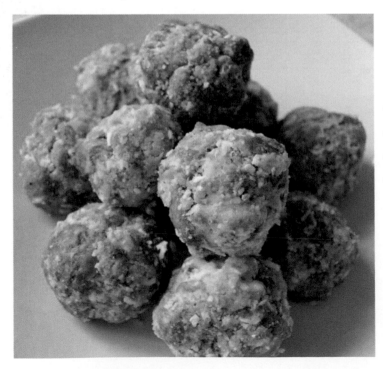

Fig and Walnut Energy Balls

Walnuts blend smooth in these sweets and the figs give crunchy goodness.

- 1½ cups / 200g **Walnuts**
- 1 cup / 150g **Dried Figs**
- 5 tbsp desiccated **Coconut**
- 1 tbsp **Cinnamon**

Place all ingredients into a food processor and blend until the mixture starts to stick together in one ball.

Roll into bite sized balls and enjoy or store in the fridge.

Did you know figs are a false fruit as they are actually a mass of inverted flowers?

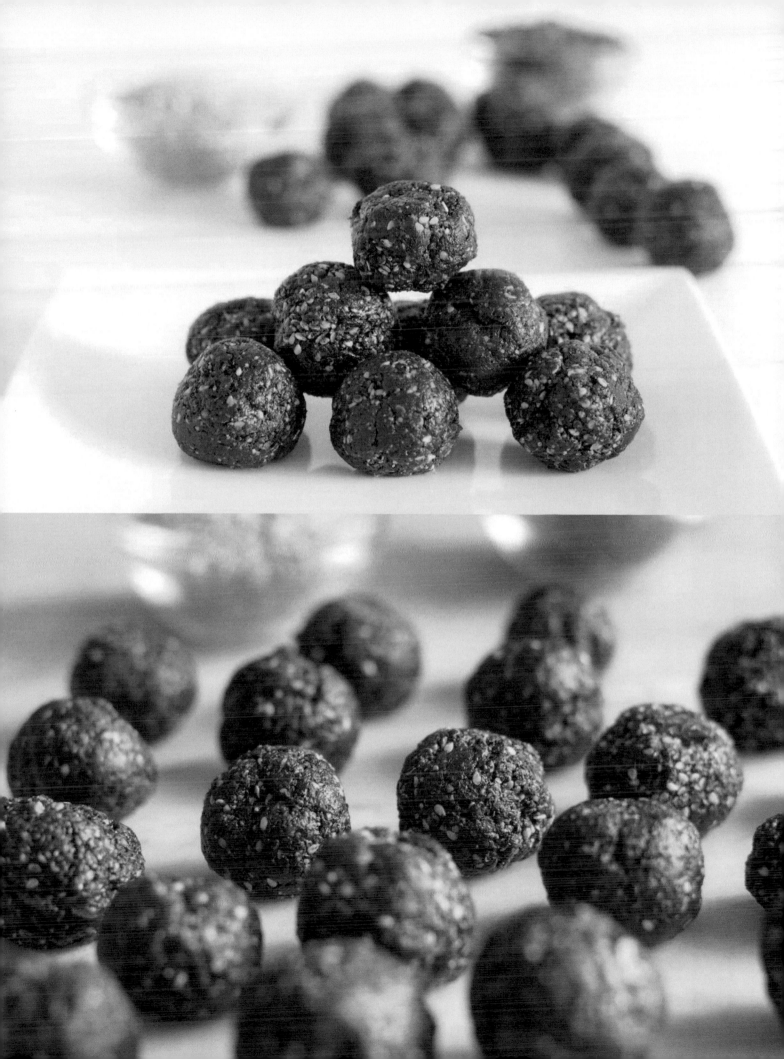

Cashew Cream Eggs

Makes 6-18 eggs | 30 mins **raw** **p**

These are much easier than they look to make and taste better than normal fondant cream eggs. It's less messy if you make half eggs and as they are quite rich, just half an egg is enough. You can wrap in foil to make one full egg. Use the raw chocolate recipe below to make raw.

Ingredients

- 4.4 oz / 125g **Chocolate**
- 1½ cups / 200g **Cashews**
- 2-6 tbsp **Maple syrup** or similar sweetener
- ⅓ cup / 80ml **Coconut oil** or **butter**
- 2-4 tbsp **Water**, just enough for blending
- 1 tsp **Vanilla**
- 1 pinch **Turmeric**
- 1 pinch **Salt**

Raw Chocolate Recipe

- ⅓ **Cacao powder**, sifted
- ⅓ **Sweetener** like maple
- ⅓ **Cacao** or **Coconut Oil** or **Butter**

To make a raw version replace the chocolate with the above recipe. Just melt the butter / oil and mix together by hand.

Equipment

- Blender, double boiler & silicon egg moulds

Method

1. Chop up the chocolate.
2. Melt 3/4 using a double boiler, remove from the heat and then add the last ¼. This is an easy way to temper the chocolate.
3. Pour 75% of the chocolate into your mould and then tilt as it dries to try to make an even coating. Keep the remaining chocolate warm to stay liquid.
4. Blend all the other ingredients together (except the turmeric) until smooth. Use a small blender jug and shake while blending.
5. Add a few more tablespoons of water if it's too thick to blend.
6. Mix a few tablespoons of the cashew cream with a pinch of turmeric to make the yellow yolk.
7. Spoon in the cashew cream and then blob on the turmeric yolk.
8. Place back in the freezer for 5 minutes.
9. Pour the remaining melted chocolate and tilt to cover.
10. Store in the fridge and enjoy within a week.

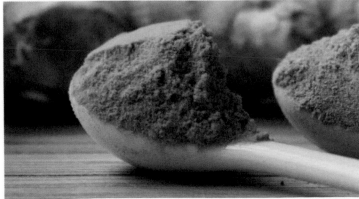

Turmeric

The "yolk" of this cream egg is coloured using turmeric. You don't taste the tiny amount in the recipe but it does add small nutritional boost.

Turmeric has lots of health benefits so I buy kilo sacks of it and add a pinch to many meals to give a nutrient and colour boost.

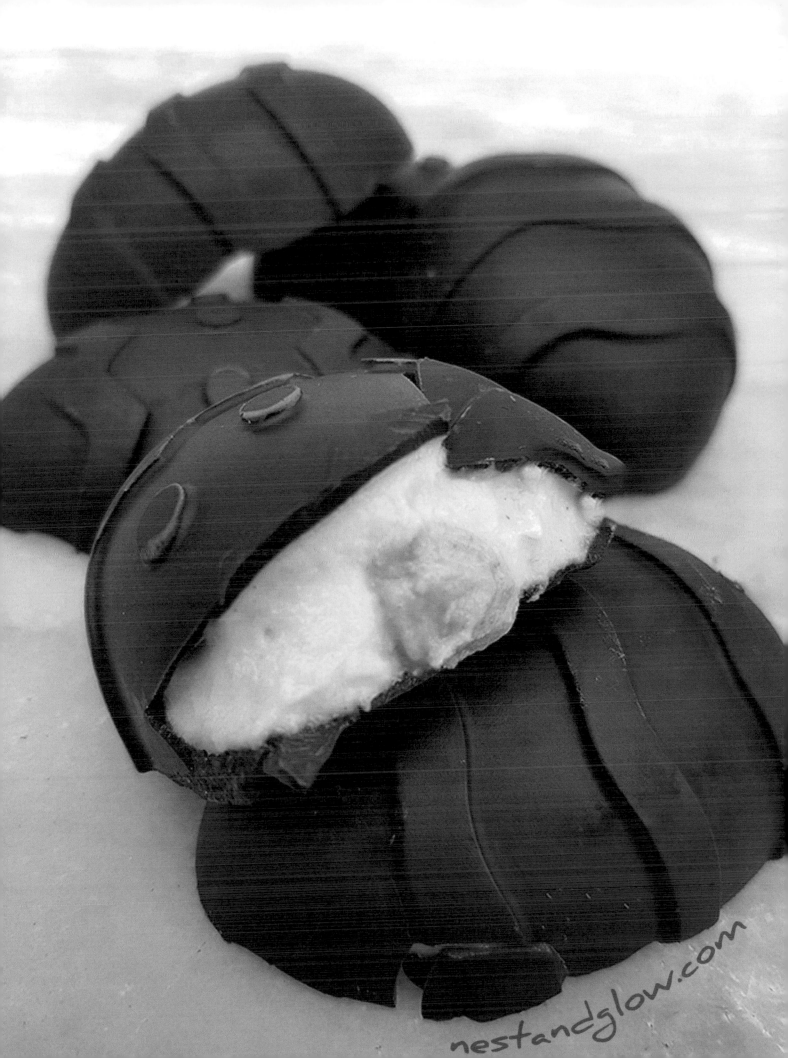

nestandglow.com

Cookie Butter Spread

Makes 1 normal sized jar | cooked 50 mins | raw 10h **raw** **nf**

This recipe is a healthy alternative cookie butter / biscuit spreads. These shop bought spreads contain wheat / gluten, refined sugar, soya, palm and other oils. This is free of all of these and is just made with seeds and sweetener.

Ingredients

- 2 cups / 280g **Sunflower seeds**
- 2 tbsp **Buckwheat**
- 4 tbsp **Maple syrup**
- 1 tsp **Vanilla**
- **Water** for soaking
- 2 pinches of **Salt**

Equipment

- Food processor
- Oven or dehydrator
- Pan
- Greaseproof paper

Method

1. Soak the sunflower seeds and buckwheat overnight in a pinch of salted water.
2. Drain the seeds then either use a dehydrator for raw or a normal oven to dry:
   - **Raw**; Spread on a dehydrator sheet and dry at 120F for 8-12 hours. Take out when bone dry.
   - **Cooked**; Spread in a pan lined with greaseproof paper and bake at 150C for about 35-35 minutes, tossing every 10 minutes to dry evenly. Take out when bone dry.
3. Place the seeds in a powerful blender and blend for minute intervals while scraping the sides down until a liquid paste is formed. This takes 4-5 minutes with a powerful blender.
4. Add the maple syrup, salt, vanilla and blend again.
5. Pour into a jar and it will last for several weeks in the fridge.

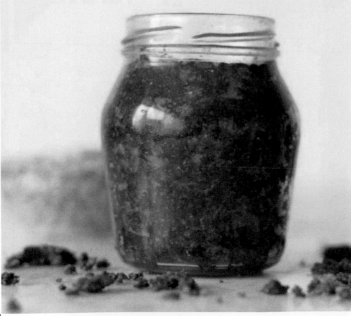

Seedtella Sunflower Chocolate Spread

To make a seed based healthy alternative to chocolate hazelnut spread use the recipe as above but replace the buckwheat with 4 tbsp of **Cocoa** or **Cacao powder**.

I use maple syrup for these two recipes to make the butter spreadable, but you can use any liquid sweetener that you like.

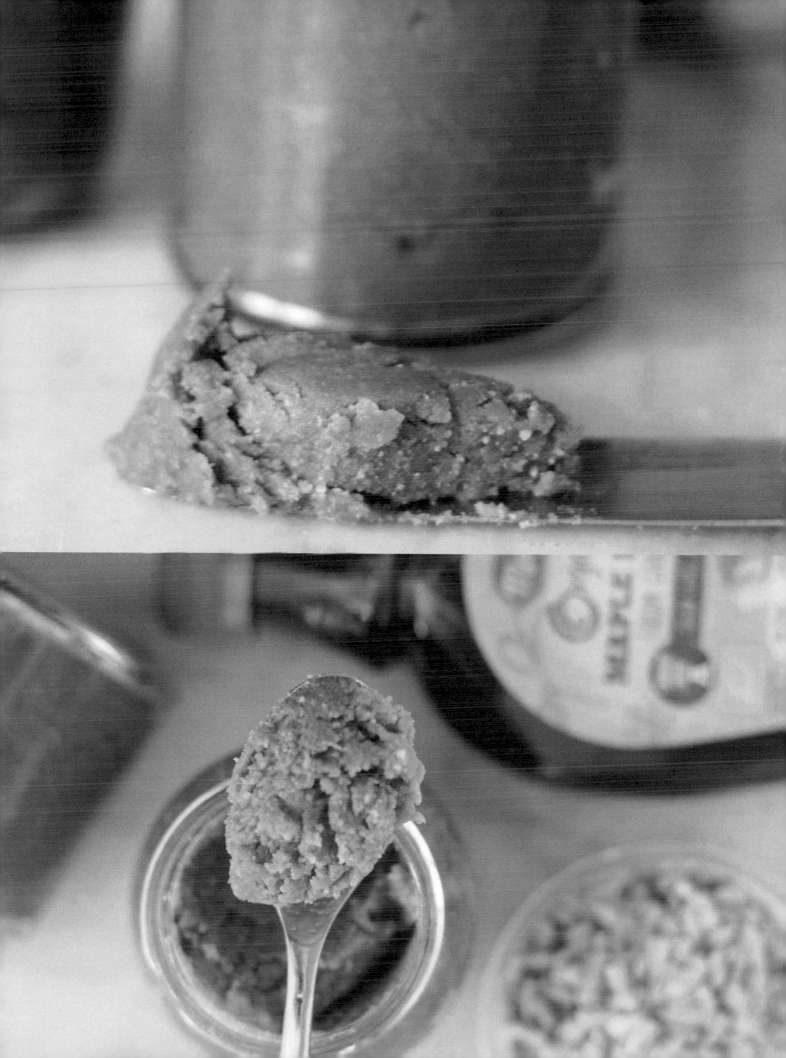

Avocado Chocolate Mint Fudge

Makes 16 large pieces | 15 mins (p) (nf)

This chocolate avocado fudge is free of dairy and full of healthy fats from avocados and coconut. If you are not a fan of mint chocolate then just leave it out to make avocado chocolate fudge. It's difficult to guess what the secret ingredient in this healthy fudge is. Other variations on this fudge are to add cinnamon or cayenne pepper.

Ingredients

- 2 large **Avocados**
- 1 can **Coconut Milk**, 15oz / 400ml
- 5 tbsp **Coconut Sugar**
- 5 tbsp **Cacao Powder**
- 2 tsp **Vanilla**
- a few drops **Peppermint extract / oil**
- ¼ tsp **Salt**
- 3 tbsp chopped **Pecans** or **Seeds** (nut free)

Equipment

- Food processor
- Greaseproof paper and Pan 8" square

Peppermint Oil

I use food grade peppermint oil for mint recipes. It's highly concentrated so just a few drops is enough. However it can be expensive and difficult to acquire so in this recipe I list peppermint extract as most shops sell it.

Method

1. Using a chilled can of coconut milk, cream off the solid coconut cream.
2. Warm your coconut cream so it is liquid and runny.
3. Place everything in the food processor apart from the pecans.
4. Blend for 2-3 minutes until it is all combined.
5. Pour into a dish lined with greaseproof paper and sprinkle with the pecan nuts.
6. Chill in the fridge overnight or 3-5 hours in the freezer then cut up.
7. Store in the fridge and enjoy within 3 days.

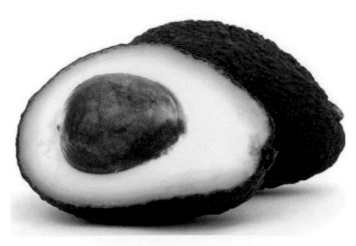

Ripening Avocados

There are many different methods people claim will speed the ripening of hard avocados but only one I've found actually works. Wrap in a paper bag with either a banana / apple / kiwi. Keep on a counter top at room temperature for 2-3 days. The gasses released by the fruit help to speed up the ripening.

Constantly buying avocados at various stages of ripeness and thinking several days in advance is almost an art-form. I sometimes worry about the amount of time "Avocado management" crosses my mind on a daily basis.

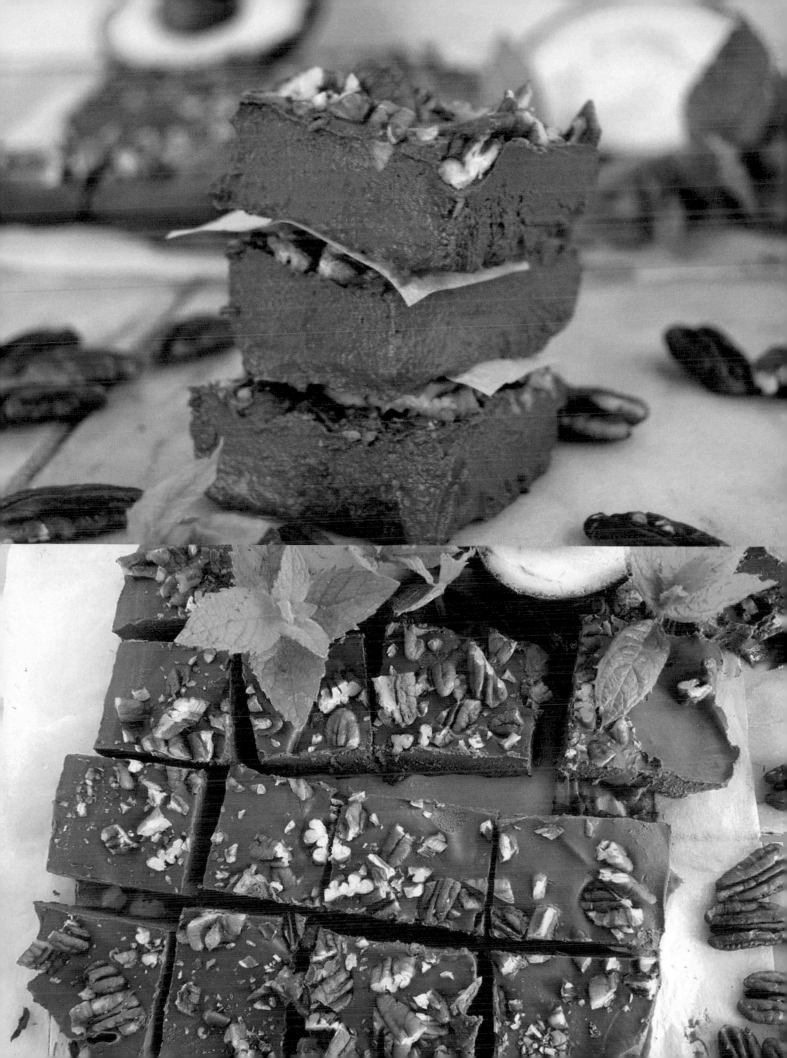

Salted Caramel Nut Chocolate Bars

Makes 24 square bars | 30 mins

These salted caramel bars are easy to make, dairy free and delicious. This is a great recipe to make with children as it doesn't involve anything hot (once the chocolate is melted) and you need to use your fingers. Even the dipping in chocolate is easy and fun.

I've decorated the ones in the photos with a few chopped up pistachios but any chopped nut on top looks great and adds texture. You can substitute the peanut butter for any other nut or seed butter. Use raw butter and chocolate to make this raw.

Ingredients

- 1 cup / 150g **Almonds**
- 1 cup / 175g **Dates**
- 4 tbsp **Peanut butter**, or any nut butter
- 2 tbsp **Maple syrup**
- 1 tsp **Sea salt**
- 1 tsp **Vanilla**
- 4.4 oz / 125g **Chocolate**
- Nuts: **Pistachios / Almonds / Hazelnuts /** any nut for decoration

Equipment

- Small blender / food processor
- Double boiler
- 6" approx square dish

Adaptation (raw)

- Use raw nut butter and a raw chocolate coating to make this raw.

Method

1. Blend together the almonds and dates until they are broken up and combined.
2. Spread the mixture in a dish using your fingers.
3. Mix together the nut butter, maple syrup, sea salt and vanilla.
4. Spread the nutty salted caramel mixture on top of the almond and date base.
5. Place in the freezer for half an hour to firm.
6. Remove from the freezer and chop into small bite size squares.
7. Melt the chocolate and chop up the nuts for the topping.
8. Hold each square with a fork over the bowl of chocolate and spoon over melted chocolate.
9. Sprinkle on the nuts while the chocolate is still liquid then put in the fridge.
10. Enjoy these salted caramel treats straight away or store in the fridge where they will stay good for a few weeks.

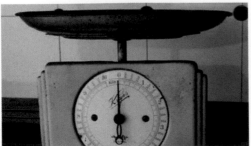

Measurements

All recipes in this book use heaped tablespoons for dry ingredients and level for liquid. Cup sizes are US, but as all recipes are full of natural products you may need to adjust to taste see "Natural Produce and Variation" on page 136.

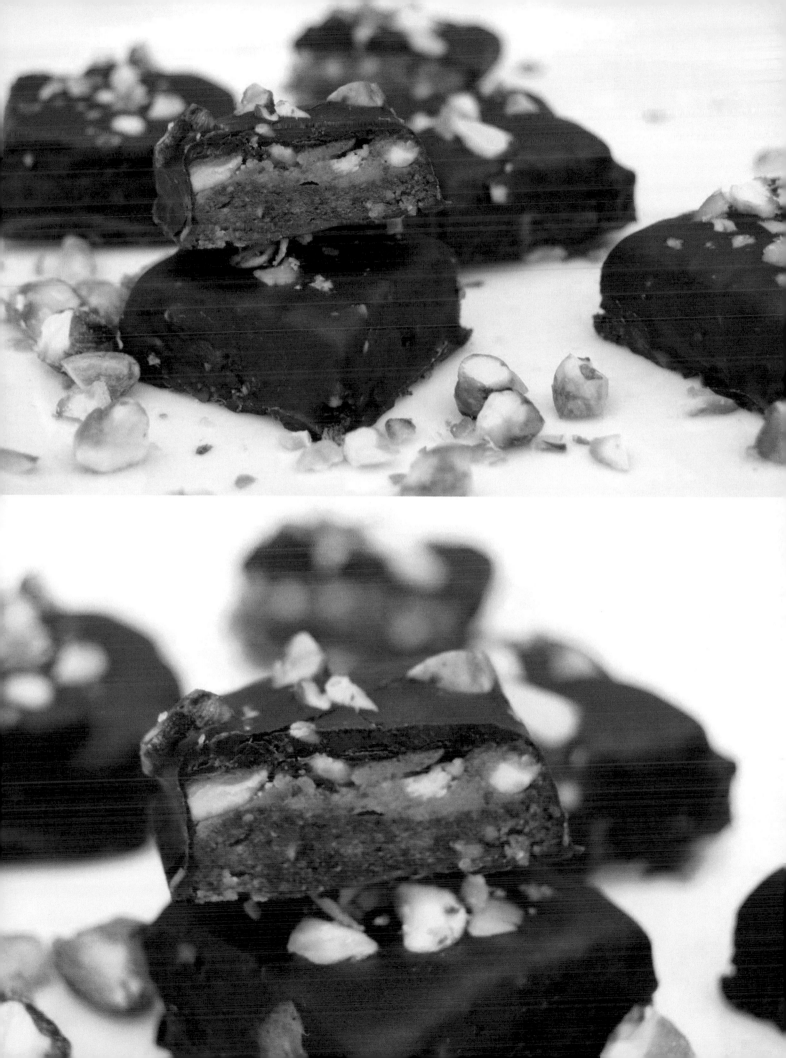

Corn Fruit Juice Sweets

Makes 60 sweets | 30 mins **p**

I've never had candy corn but I have a fascination with making a healthy version of junk food. These use orange, carrot and pineapple juice along with cashew nuts to make a candy full of good stuff. Many people that don't like candy corn have liked this juice and nut alternative.

Ingredients

- 2 tbsp **Cashew nuts**
- 3-6 tbsp **Maple syrup** / date syrup / any liquid sweetener
- 4½ tsp **Agar Agar Powder** (page 94)
- 1 tsp **Vanilla extract**
- ½ cup / 120ml **Orange juice**
- ½ cup / 120ml **Carrot juice**
- 1 cup / 240ml **Pineapple Juice**

Equipment

- Blender
- Pan
- Dish 6" by 4"

Method

1. Into a blender jug add the cashew nuts, 1-2 tbsp of your sweetener, the vanilla and a cup / 240 ml of water. Blend until smooth.
2. Pour the cashew mixture into a pan, add 1½ tsp of agar agar and simmer for 5 minutes on a low heat. Stir constantly to stop the bottom from burning.
3. Let the cashew mixture cool for 5 minutes and pour into a dish that's about 6" by 4". Then place in the freezer.
4. Add the orange and carrot juice into a pan with 1-2 tbsp maple syrup, 1½ tsp of agar agar and bring to a boil then simmer for 5 minutes.
5. Let the orange mixture cool for 5 minutes then pour on top of the cashew layer in the dish and place back in the freezer.
6. Repeat steps 4-5 for the pineapple juice.
7. The mixture should be set after 15 minutes in the freezer.
8. Push the sweet mixture out of the dish and then slice length ways.
9. Cut each slice into triangles and they are ready to eat.
10. Store in the fridge and eat within 3 days as they contain fruit juice.

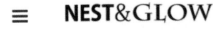

≡ **NEST&GLOW** Q

——— LEAVE A COMMENT ———

Your Comment

Questions or Help

If you have any questions or need any help simply search for "<recipe name> nest and glow" and you will find the relevant page on nestandglow.com. There you may find your question is answered in the comments or you can write a new comment and I'll reply.

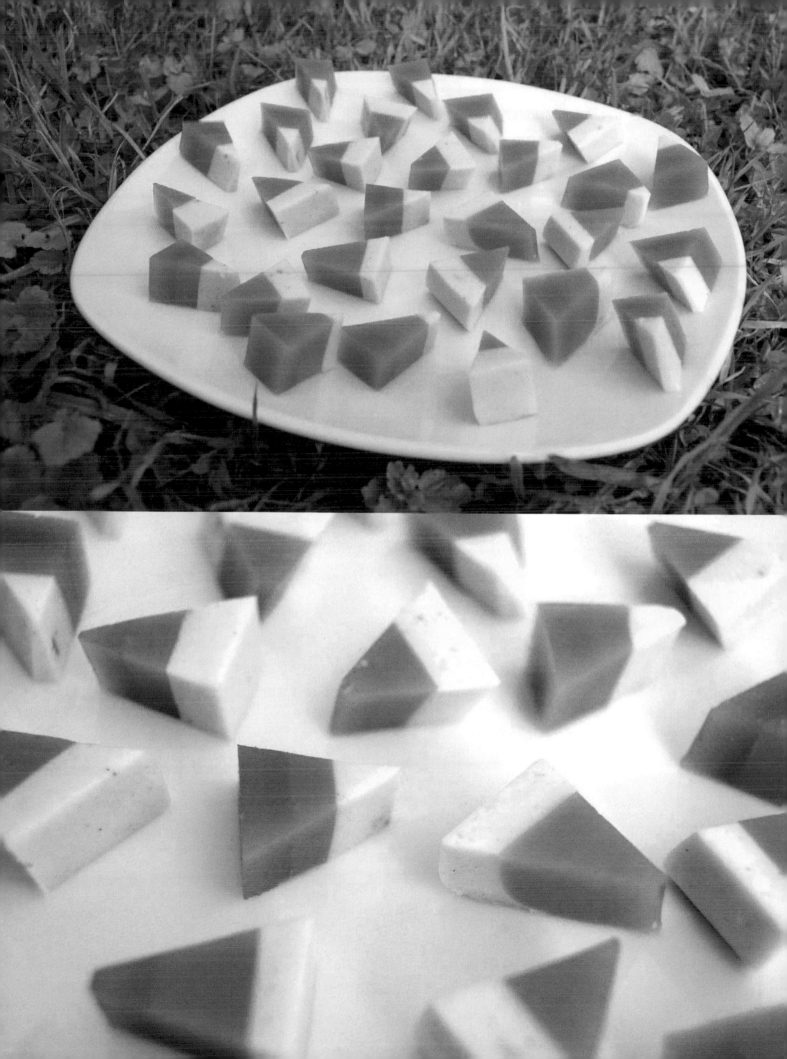

Ginger Turmeric Vanilla Cookies

Makes 8 cookies | 45 mins

These golden ginger turmeric cookies are quick and simple to make. You can ice them with the cashew vanilla icing if you like but they are great without. The same combination of oats and bananas can make many different types of healthy cookies.

Cookie ingredients

- 3 **Bananas**
- 1½ cups / 200g ground **Oats**
- 2 tbsp ground **Ginger**
- 1 tbsp **Turmeric**
- pinch of **Salt** and **Pepper**

Equipment

- Oven and Baking tray
- Greaseproof / parchment paper

Cashew Vanilla Icing

- ¾ cup / 115g **Cashew nuts**
- 2 tbsp **Sweetener** such as Maple syrup
- 1 tsp **Vanilla**
- 2 tbsp **Coconut oil**, optional – substitute with extra water
- a splash of **Water** for blending
- a sprinkle of **Turmeric** or **Ginger** to top

Method

1. Mix all of the dry cookie ingredients together.
2. Mash the bananas with a fork and then mix with the dry ingredients.
3. Spoon onto a baking tray, try to make about 8 the same size and a roughly round shape.
4. Bake at 180C / 350F for 12 / 15 minutes until they start to get a bit of colour. You will smell a banana caramel smell when they are cooked.
5. Blend all of the cashew vanilla icing ingredients together.
6. Place in the freezer for 5 minutes to firm.
7. Ice the cookies and then sprinkle with a pinch of turmeric or ginger.
8. Keep in an airtight container in the fridge and enjoy within three days.

Banana Oat Cookies

You can use the recipe of 3 bananas and 1½ cups / 200g ground Oats to make all of these;

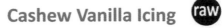

| Cranberry Cacao | Raisin | Giant Chocolate | Pumpkin Spice |

All the recipes for the above cookies are at nestandglow.com - but they are easy to workout.

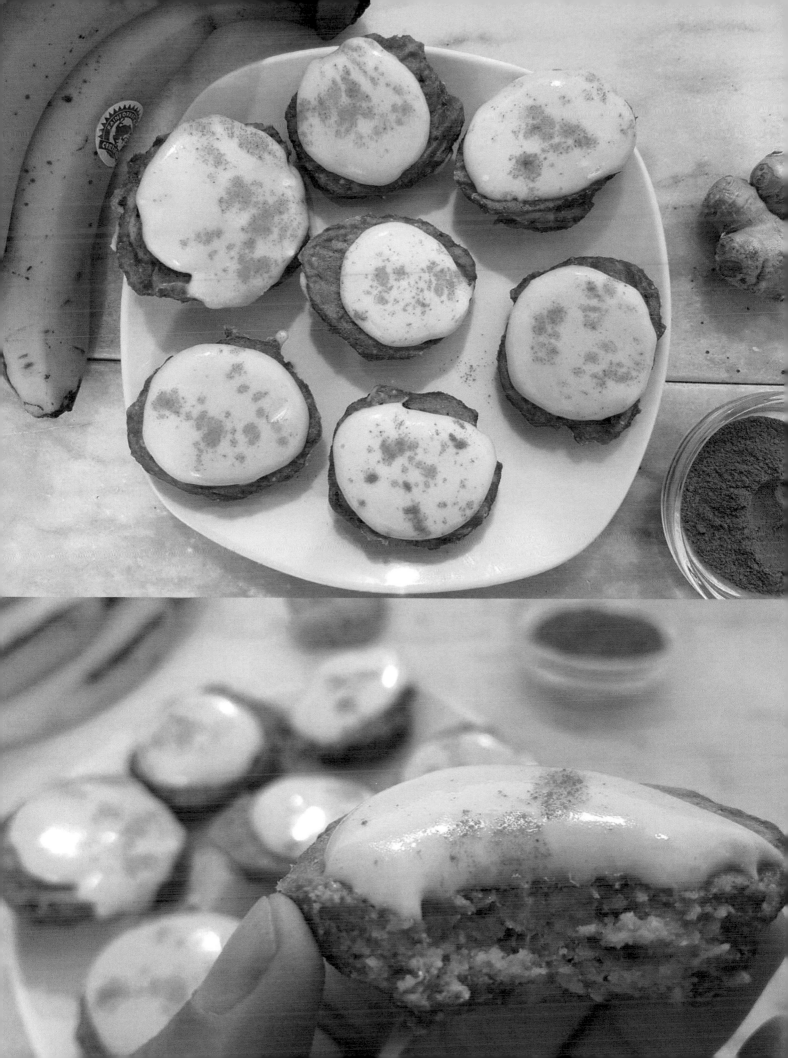

Chocolate Fudge Mung Bean Brownies

Makes 9 large brownies | 1h 20 mins

These healthy chocolate fudge mung bean brownies have no flour, eggs or butter and are 100% plant based. People regularly call them the best brownies ever. Chocolate chunks sprinkled on top give a rustic home baked look that I love.

Ingredients

- 1½ cups / 300g cooked **Mung beans** (1 tin)
- 3 tbsp **Cocoa powder**
- ½ cup / 40g ground **Oats**
- 4 tbsp **Maple syrup** / date syrup / or any sweetener
- 6-8 pitted **Dates**
- 2 tbsp melted **Coconut oil / butter**, optional
- 2 tsp **Vanilla extract**
- ½ cup / 90g of **Chocolate chips** / chunks
- ½ tsp **Baking powder**
- pinch of **Salt**
- 2 tbsp **Chocolate chips** / chunks to top

Equipment

- Food processor / blender
- 8" Baking pan, Greaseproof paper and Oven

Method

1. Preheat the oven to 350F / 180C.
2. Place everything apart from the chocolate chips / chunks in a food processor and blend until smooth. You can use a blender if you don't have a food processor but it will need to be blended in batches.
3. Stir in the chocolate chips / chunks and then spread out in a 8" pan. I use a silicon pan so they pop out easily, if using a metal pan you will need to place some greaseproof paper inside.
4. Bake in the oven for 16-20 minutes until a knife comes out clean.
5. Take out of the oven, sprinkle on 2 tbsp of chocolate chips and leave for 15 minutes to cool before removing from the pan.
6. Pop out of the pan and slice into about 9 brownies.
7. They are best enjoyed still warm and gooey but will last a few days in the fridge. It's best to re-heat if eating from the fridge.

Pressure Cooker

I often use a stove top pressure cooker to cook my beans and pulses from dry. This saves money, excess packaging and transport costs. Pressure cookers may seem daunting with the high pressure steam released and the possibility of exploding. However once you learn to use one you will find it invaluable for making healthy and inexpensive plant based food quickly.

There are modern pressure cookers that don't use the stove and are apparently fool-proof to use but I haven't used one as my pressure cooker bought 15 years ago as an impulse buy is still in perfect working condition.

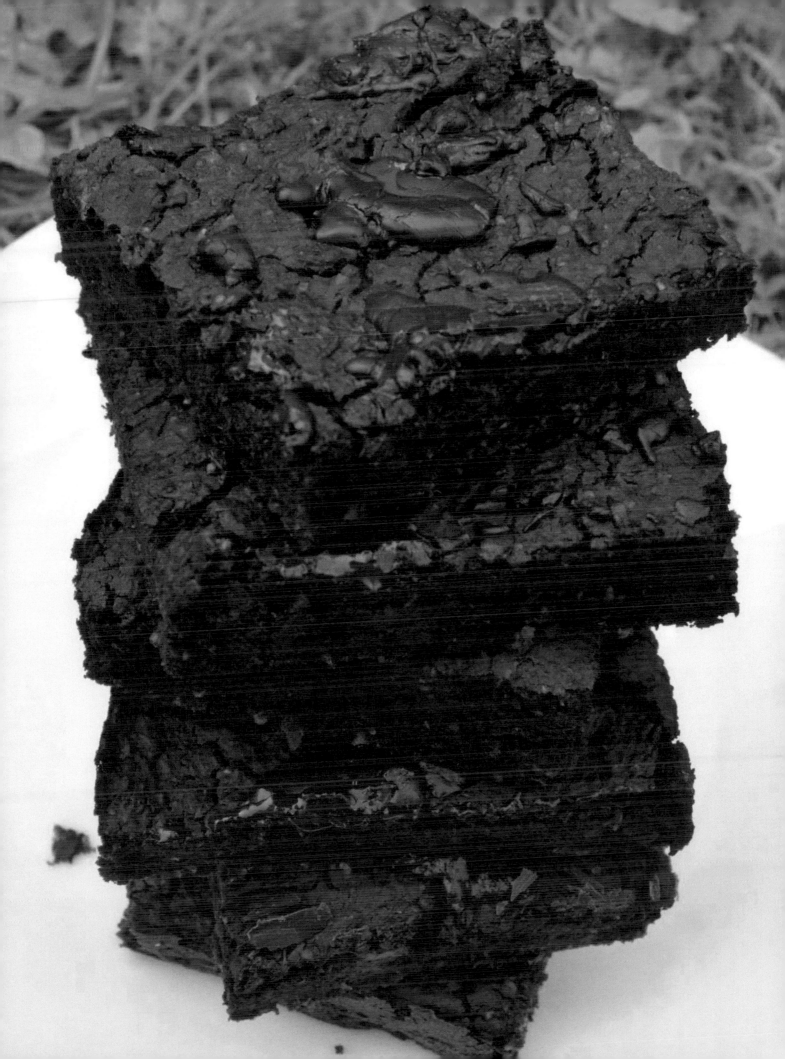

Quinoa Chocolate Banana Bread

Makes 9 slices | 1h 20 mins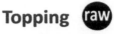

Sweet banana bread with a dark deep chocolate taste. Sweetened purely with fruit and high in protein. A slice of this is a substantial and filling snack.

Ingredients

- 2 **Bananas**
- 1 cup / 180g **Quinoa**, soaked overnight
- ½ cup / 75g **Raisins**
- ½ cup / 50g **Cocoa / Cacao powder**
- ½ cup / 50g **Desiccated Coconut**
- ½ tsp **Baking powder**
- 3 tbsp **Chia seeds**, soaked in 9 tbsp **Water**
- pinch of **Salt**
- 1 cup **Water**

Topping (raw)

- 2 **Bananas**
- 2 tbsp **Cocoa / Cacao powder**
- 2 tbsp **Nuts or seeds**, chopped

Equipment

- Food processor / blender
- Oven
- Square tin about 8"
- Greaseproof paper

Method

1. Soak the quinoa the night before, then drain and rinse.
2. Soak the ground chia seeds while adding everything for the banana bread into a blender then add the chia last.
3. Blend smooth and pour into a greaseproof paper lined tin.
4. Bake for an hour at 190C / 375F until a knife comes out mostly clean.
5. Leave to cool and firm while you make the icing. It will firm up as it cools.
6. Mash two bananas with 2 tbsp of cacao powder.
7. Spread the icing on the cooled cake and top with chopped nuts or seeds.
8. Enjoy within 3 days and keep in the fridge.

Notes

Overripe bananas that are almost too soft to eat are perfect for this recipe as they are super sweet, soft and fluffy. It's the perfect recipe to use up bananas.

This base recipe is nut-free but I just love hazelnuts and chocolate so couldn't resist sprinkling a few chopped on top. These are totally optional and can be replaced with seeds such as sunflower or shredded coconut if you prefer. I've listed the recipe as nut free as the only nuts are the optional garnish.

The basic recipe is for a rich cacao slightly bitter chocolate bread. If you want it sweeter then double the amount of raisins or add some liquid sweetener. I like my dark chocolate, so just use half a cup of raisins, but for non-dark chocolate lovers you will want to add some more sweetness.

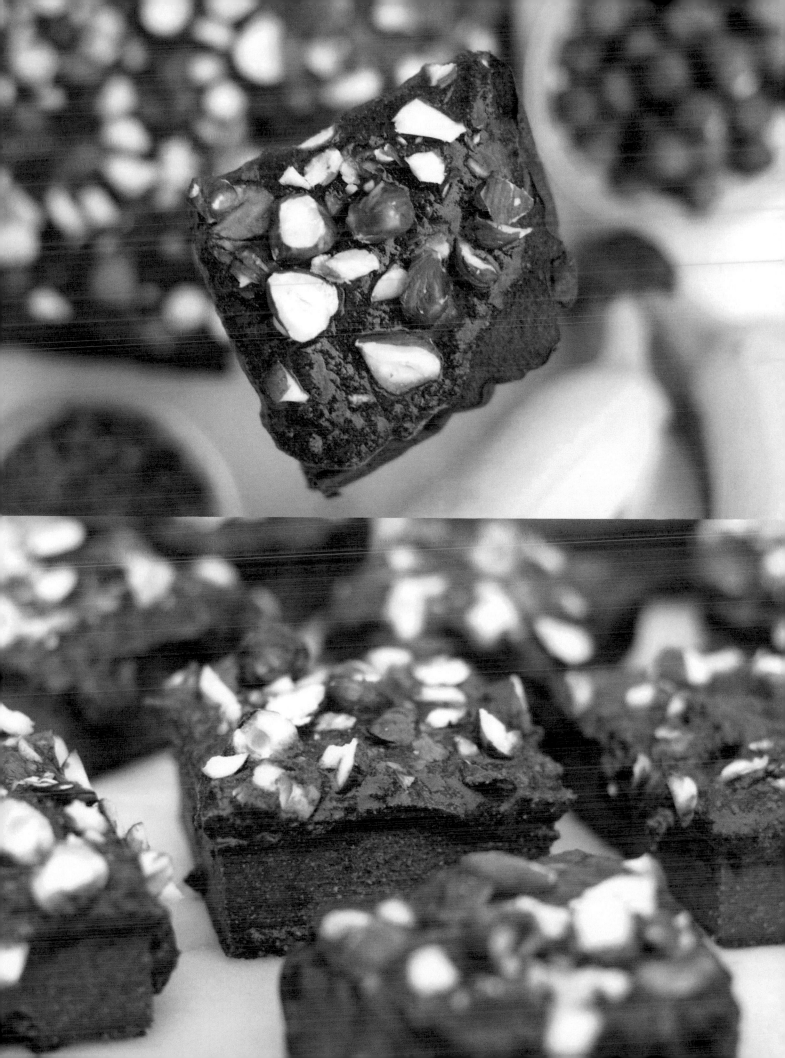

Black Bean Chocolate Fudge Muffins with Vanilla Frosting

Makes 6 muffins | 45 mins

The recipe is very simple and even if you're not good at baking, like me, it's hard to go wrong with making these. If you are testing these out on others don't tell them the special ingredient until after they have tried them. Loaded with nutrients, vitamins, fibre, protein and heart-healthy fats.

Muffins

- 1 tin / 240g cooked **Black beans**
- 3 tbsp **Cocoa powder**
- ½ cup / 40g ground **Oats**
- 2-4 tbsp **Maple syrup** / date syrup or any sweetener
- 6-8 pitted **Dates**
- 2 tbsp melted **Coconut butter** or **oil**
- 2 tsp **Vanilla** extract
- ½ cup / 80g **Chocolate chips** /chunks
- ½ tsp **Baking powder**
- pinch of **Salt**

Cashew Vanilla Frosting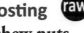

- ¾ cup / 100g **Cashew nuts**
- 2 tbsp melted **Coconut butter / oil**
- 1 tbsp **Maple syrup** / date syrup / or any sweetener
- 1 tsp **Vanilla extract**
- 2-4 tbsp **Water**, just enough for blending

Equipment

- Food processor
- Muffin tin
- Muffin cases - paper or silicon
- Oven

Method

1. Preheat the oven to 350F / 180C.
2. Place everything for the muffins apart from the chocolate chips / chunks in a food processor and blend until smooth. You can use a blender if you don't have a food processor but it will need to be blended in batches.
3. Stir in the chocolate chips / chunks and then spoon into a lined muffin pan.
4. Bake in the oven for 16-20 minutes until a knife comes out clean.
5. Blend all the frosting ingredients together then place in the freezer for 5 minutes. It should then be a consistency where it doesn't pour but is still spreadable. If the frosting is too runny, stir in some more melted coconut oil and chill.
6. Spread the icing on top of the muffins. Garnish with some chocolate shavings.
7. They are delicious while warm and gooey but still taste amazing cold and will last a few days in the fridge.

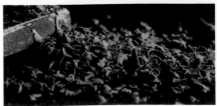

Chocolate

I always use a very dark chocolate for the recipes in this book. Usually one that is 85% cocoa or higher. Very dark chocolate is low in sugar, high in depth of flavour and full of nutrients.

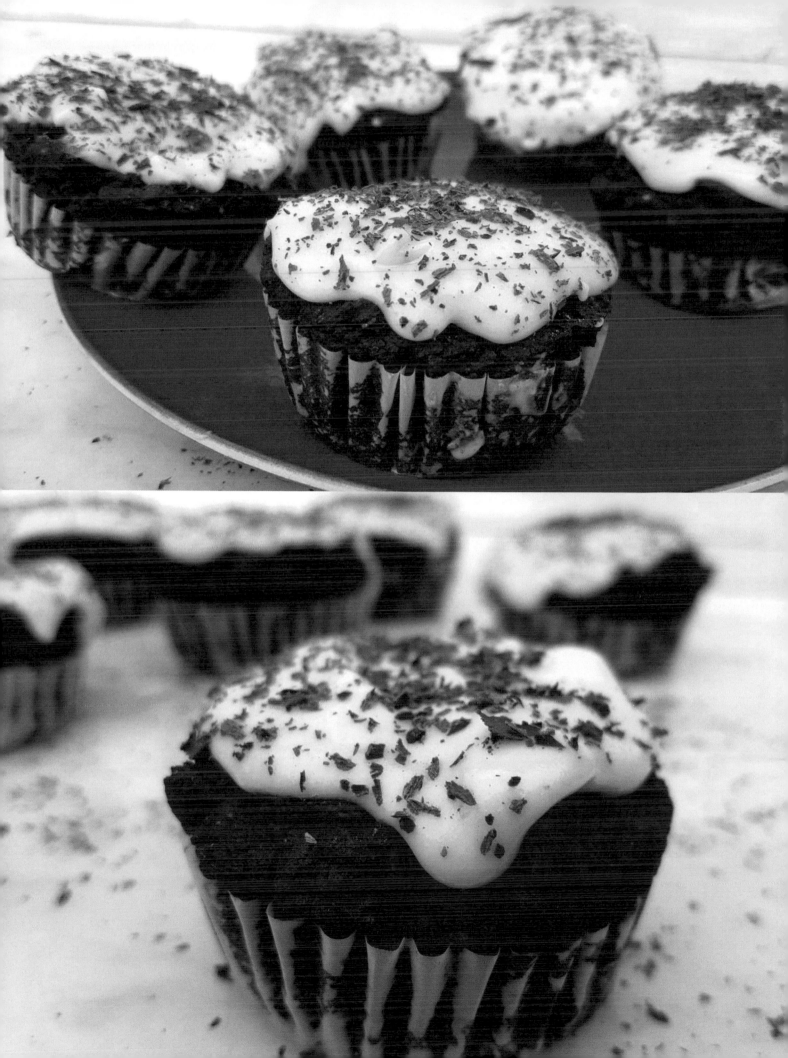

Banana Cinnamon Roll Buns

Single bun | 2h 10 mins cooked | 12h raw **raw** **p** **nf**

These easy to make cinnamon roll buns are just made of fruit and spices. For this recipe you can either bake in the oven or if you have a dehydrator make the raw version. The raw version does take 6 times longer to make.

Ingredients per cinnamon bun

- 1 **Banana**
- 1 tsp **Cinnamon**
- 1 tbsp **Dates**
- 1 drop of **Vanilla extract**

Equipment

- Food processor / small blender
- Oven for baked
- Dehydrator for raw
- Greaseproof paper

Method

1. Cut each banana length ways into thirds. Don't worry if some of the bananas break up – just use these for the inner part.
2. Place onto a non stick sheet so that they will peal off easily.
3. Either bake for an hour at 250F / 120C or dehydrate for 6 hours at 100F / 40C.
4. Blend the dates with vanilla and a touch of water to make the date paste.
5. Take one dried banana slice and place on a flat surface.
6. Spread on the date paste, sprinkle with cinnamon, repeat this then roll up into a tight bun.
7. Then either bake for an hour at 250F / 120C or dehydrate for 6 hours at 100F / 40C.
8. Enjoy immediately or keep in the fridge and consume within a few days.

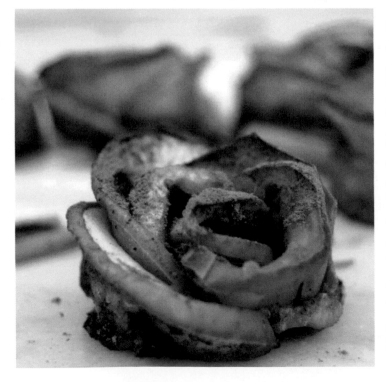

Apple Roses

These apple roses are a fun enhancement to the banana cinnamon buns recipe.

Ingredients

3 **bananas**, 3 **apples**, 3 tbsp **dates**, 3 tbsp **raisins**, 3 tbsp **cinnamon**, 2 cups / 500ml water

Method - Steps 1-3 above then:

Core and thinly slice all the apples.

Blend the dates, raisins and water.

Simmer the sliced apples in the blended fruit water for 5 minutes until softened.

Roll the apple slices inside the bananas then bake or dehydrate as per step 7.

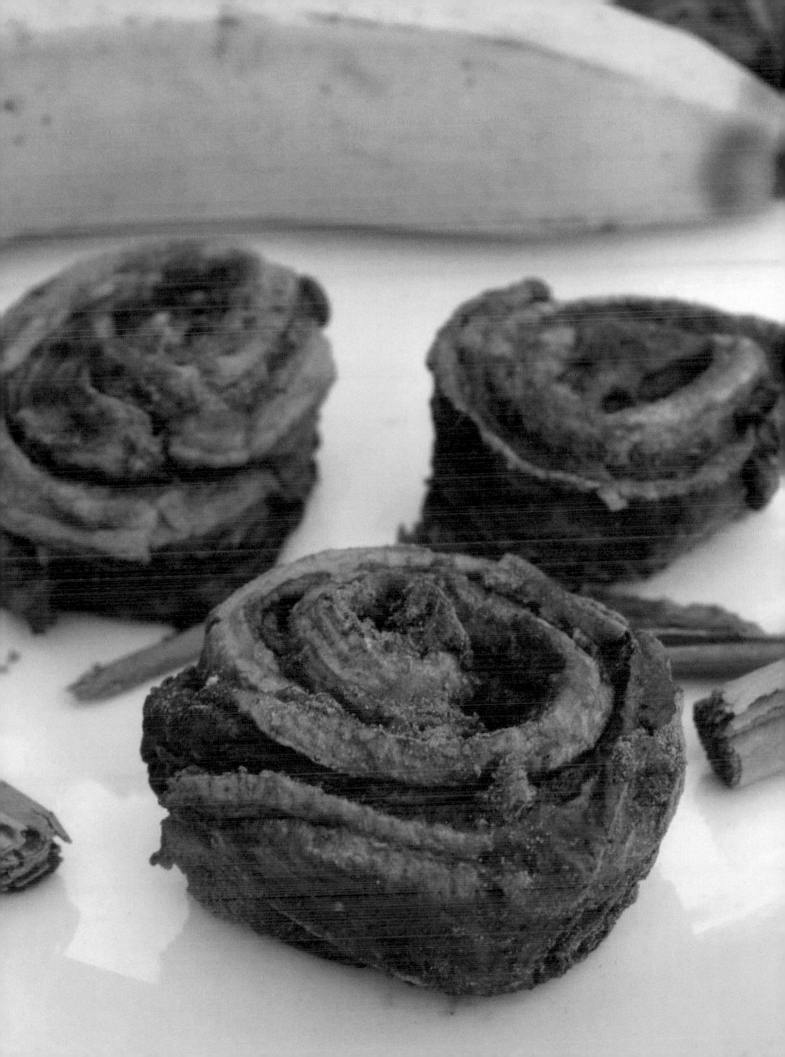

Banana Coconut Macaroons

Makes 16 macaroons | 30 mins (raw) (p) (nf)

Easy and fun macaroons that are sweetened just with banana. You can make these as either raw or baked. In the photo I made baked ones to make this recipe accessible to all.

Ingredients

- 2 **Bananas**
- 1¼ cups / 125g **Desiccated coconut**
- 3.5oz / 100g **Dark** or **Raw chocolate**

Equipment

- Fork
- Oven / Dehydrator
- Greaseproof paper

Method

1. Peel and mash the very ripe bananas.
2. Mix in the coconut with the mashed bananas, I find using your hands easiest.
3. Spoon a heaped tablespoon of the mixture and roll into a ball then flatten.
4. **Cooked**; bake at 350F / 180C for about 15 minutes until they start to go golden.
5. **Raw**; dehydrate for 6 hours at 110F then flip and dehydrate for 4 more hours.
6. Leave to cool while melting the chocolate.
7. Dip into the chocolate then place on greaseproof paper to cool.
8. Store in the fridge and enjoy within 3 days. You can also store in the freezer for up to 3 months and defrost at room temperature.

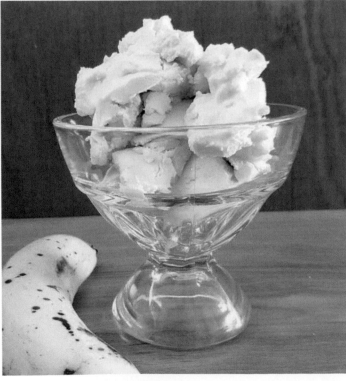

Banana Coconut Ice-cream

Many dairy-free healthy ice creams are either banana or coconut. Both are good; sometimes you fancy a pure fruit banana ice-cream and other times a creamy coconut ice-cream. When you want something in between try this!

Serves 2 | 5 minutes

- 2 frozen **Bananas**, peeled
- ½ cup / 50g desiccated **Coconut**
- 1 tsp **Vanilla**
- ½ cup / 120ml **water**

Blend coconut and water in small jug until smooth, then add everything else, blend more and enjoy.

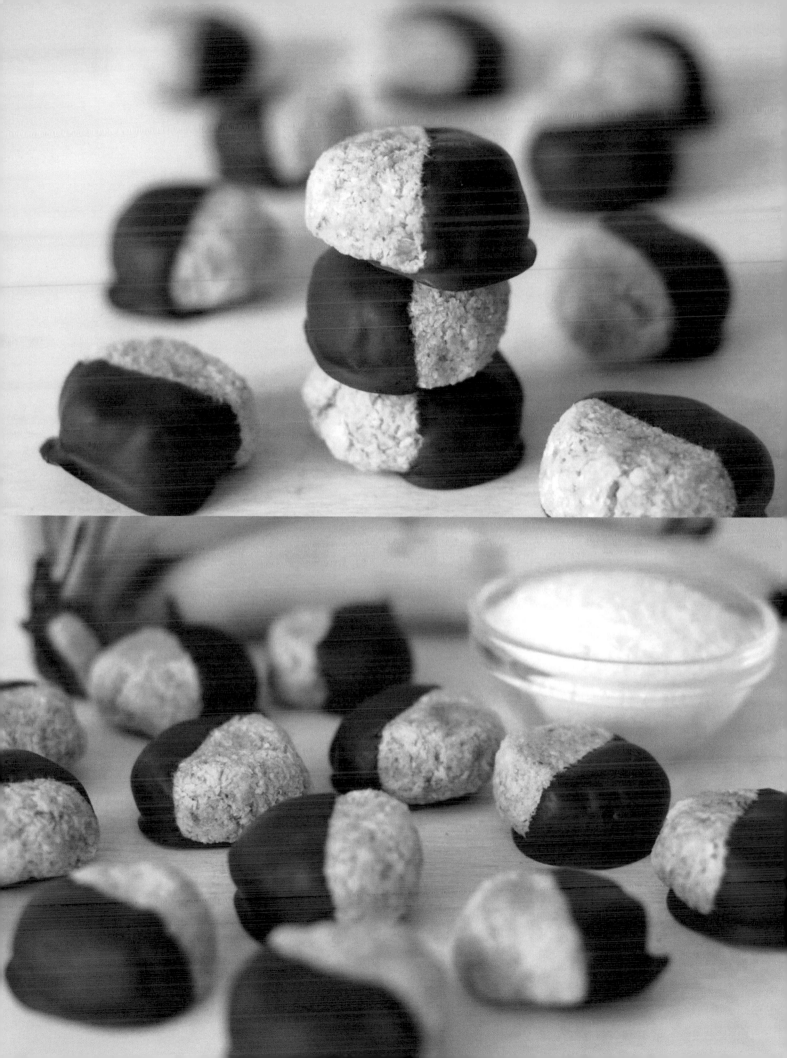

Chocolate Chip Almond Chickpea Blondies

Makes 26 Blondies | 45 mins

Moist and fudgy just like a normal blondie and you wouldn't even realise how healthy they are from how good they taste. Bursting with nutrition, heart-healthy fats and fibre. Remember to use gluten-free oats if you are sensitive to gluten, see "Oats and Gluten" on page 80.

Ingredients

- 1 can **Chickpeas**, 15oz / 400ml
- ½ cup / 70g **Almonds**
- ½ cup / 90g **Chocolate chips**
- ¾ cup / 140g **Dates**
- 1 cup / 90g rolled **Oats**, ground
- 2-4 tbsp **Maple / Coconut syrup** or any other sweetener
- 2 tbsp **Coconut oil / butter**, optional
- 2 tsp **Vanilla**
- ½ tsp **Baking powder**
- a pinch of **Salt**
- a few tbsp of **Water**, just enough to blend to a smooth batter

Equipment

- Food processor
- Oven
- 10" approx square dish
- Greaseproof / parchment paper

Method

1. Preheat the oven to 350F / 180C.
2. Melt the coconut and grind the oats.
3. Add everything apart from the water and chocolate to a food processor. Blend until smooth adding water a tablespoon at a time.
4. Stir in most of the chocolate chips and spread in the pan lined with greaseproof paper.
5. Bake for 25-30 minutes until they are slightly golden. Add a few more chocolate chips on the top once taken out of the oven.
6. Allow to cool and then cut into slices.

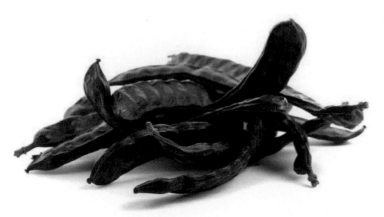

Carob

If you are looking for a caffeine free alternative to chocolate / cacao then try carob. You can buy it in bars, powder or pods.

Carob doesn't quite have the same depth of flavour as chocolate but is a useful alternative with various health benefits.

Chewing on a whole unprocessed carob pod is a tasty on the go snack - just look out for the seeds.

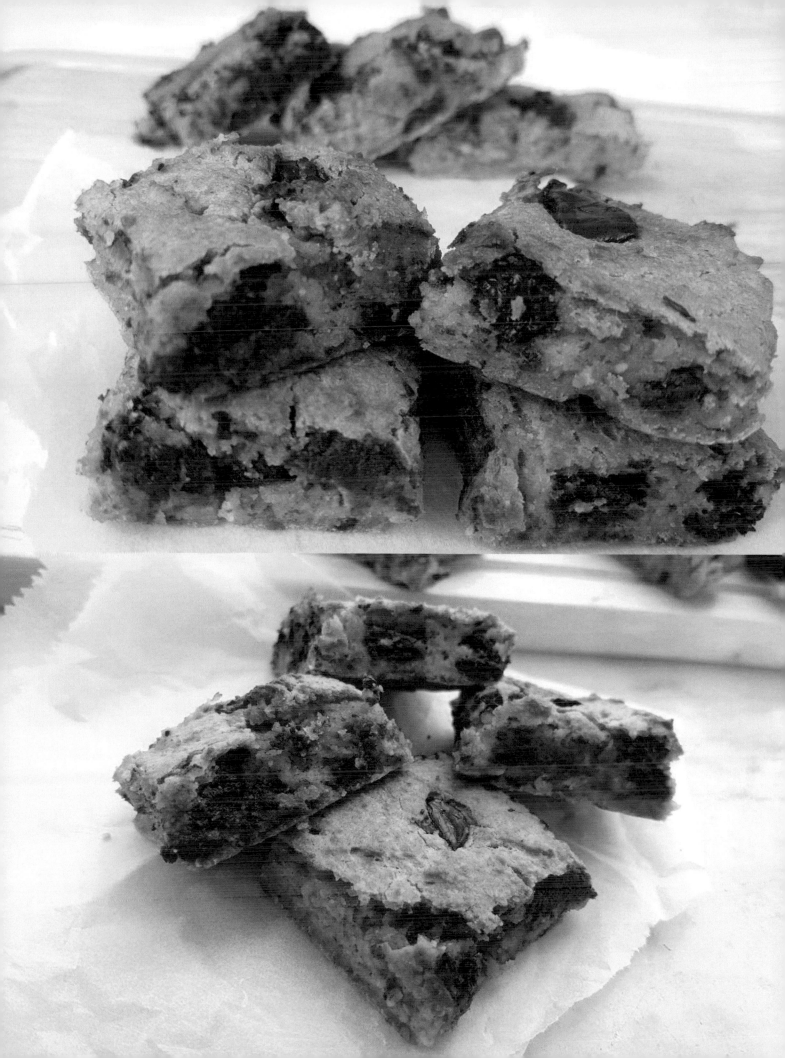

Chocolate Ultimate Brownie

Serves 8 | 10 mins 🅿 🆖

These brownies with sweet potato, avocado frosting, coconut whipped cream and sunflower seed caramel are what I confidently call the ultimate healthy chocolate fudge brownie!

Brownie Mixture

- 2 lb / 1kg **Sweet potato**
- 1 cup / 140g **Sunflower seeds**, soaked
- 1 cup / 175g **Dates**
- 1 cup / 120g **Buckwheat** or **Coconut flour (P)**
- 4 tbsp **Cacao / Cocoa powder**
- 4 tbsp **Maple / Coconut syrup**, or similar
- 3 tbsp **Chia seeds** soaked in 9 tbsp **Water**
- 2 tsp **Cinnamon**
- a pinch of **Salt**

Avocado Chocolate Frosting

- 2 **Avocados**
- 4-6 tbsp **Maple / Coconut syrup**
- 4 tbsp **Cacao / Cocoa powder**

Coconut Whipped Cream

- ½ can **Coconut milk**, full fat

Chocolate sauce

- 1 tbsp **Cacao / Cocoa powder**
- 1 tbsp **Maple syrup**
- 1 tbsp **Water**

Sunflower caramel

- 2 tbsp **Sunflower seeds**, soaked
- 2 tbsp **Coconut sugar**
- 6 tbsp **Water**

Equipment

- Food processor / small blender
- Oven
- Greaseproof paper & Tin

Method

1. Bake the sweet potatoes for about half an hour at 350F / 180C until soft. Allow to cool then peel away the skin so you are left with just the flesh.
2. Soak the chia seeds in 9 tbsp of water.
3. Soak the sunflower seeds for at least 10 minutes then rinse and drain.
4. Place all of the brownie ingredients into a food processor for 2-3 minutes until broken up.
5. Pour the brownie mixture into a tin lined with greaseproof paper. Use a large tin about 8" by 8", any will do but you may need to adjust the cooking times.
6. Bake at 180C / 350F for 30-35 minutes until a fork comes out clean. Leave to cool and firm up for 15 minutes before taking out of the pan.
7. Blend all the avocado frosting ingredients together, you may need to add a few tbsp of water.
8. Whip the coconut milk for a minute to make the coconut whipped cream.
9. Blend all the sunflower caramel ingredients together to make this nut free caramel sauce.
10. Layer up the treat; brownie layer followed by avocado frosting, repeat this twice then top with coconut whipped cream and drizzle with chocolate sauce and sunflower seed caramel.
11. It looks best with three layers of brownies, but it will self-destruct into a delicious mess when you attempt to tackle it!

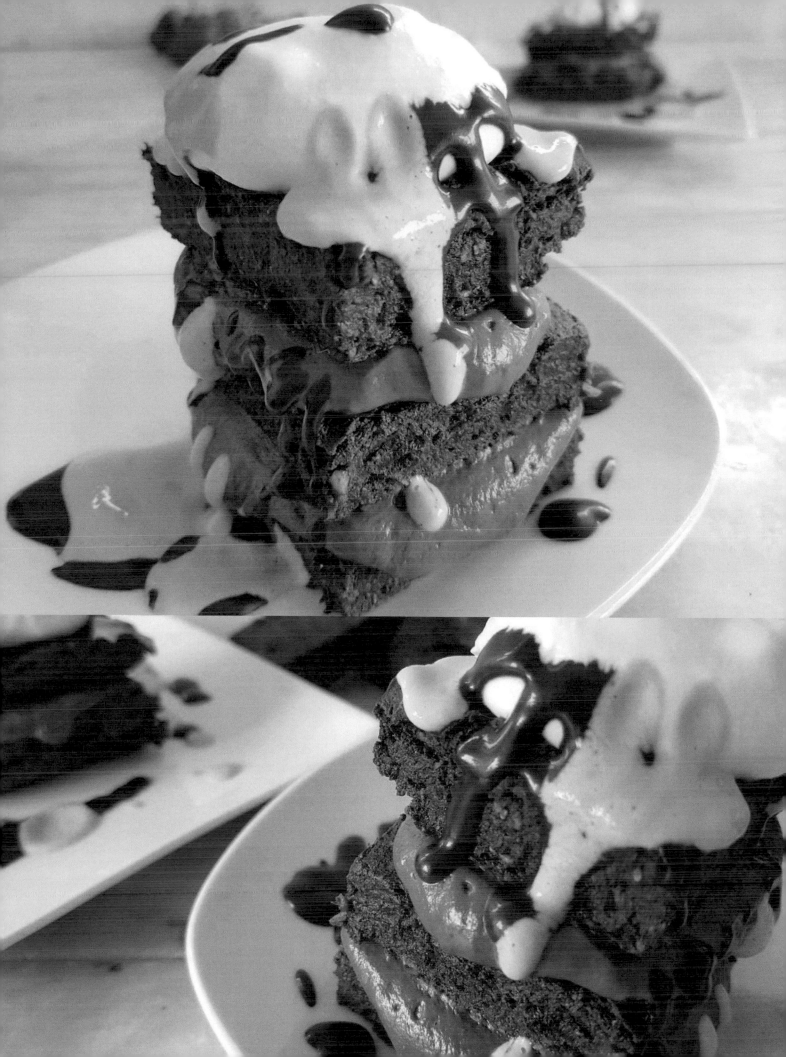

Mango Lime Chia Almond Pudding

Makes 4 puddings | 10 mins (raw) (p) (nf)

Chia puddings are an excellent food to make in advance and grab when you're on the go. This mango Lime Chia Almond Pudding is easy to make, lasts for a couple of days and keeps you full for hours. The sweetness of the mango is mixed with zesty lime for a tangy sweet topping.

Ingredients

- 2 cups / 500ml **Plant milk,** like almond
- ½ cup / 80g **Chia seeds**
- 2 tbsp **Maple syrup**, or any other sweetener
- 1 tsp **Vanilla**
- 1 medium **Mango**
- 1 **Lime** juiced

Equipment

- Blender
- Whisk or Fork
- Pots

Notes

- Use seed milk for nut free

Method

1. Mix the milk, maple syrup and vanilla together.
2. Whisk by hand the chia seeds and leave 20 minutes to gel up. Make sure there are no clumps of chia.
3. Blend together the mango flesh and lime juice.
4. Pour out the chia mixture into 4 pots and then top with the mango lime coulis.
5. Store in the fridge and they will last for a couple of days.

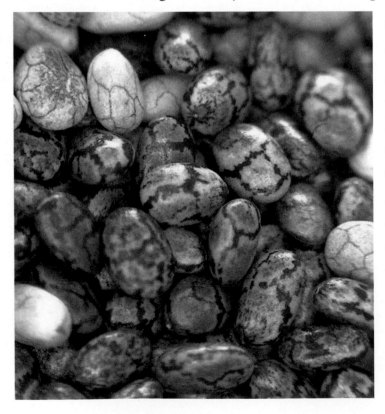

Chia Seeds

These little seeds almost look like prehistoric eggs when magnified. They originate from central and South America where the Aztecs and Mayans apparently used these nutrient dense seeds for energy.

They are high in fibre so help keep you fuller for longer, contain 17% protein and all 9 essential amino acids. Also provide a source of calcium and magnesium.

When soaked in a liquid they absorb ten times their volume to become a gel. This gel is said to give endurance benefits but can also be used as an egg replacement in many recipes. Soaked chia seeds throughout this book are used in baked goodies to help give structure.

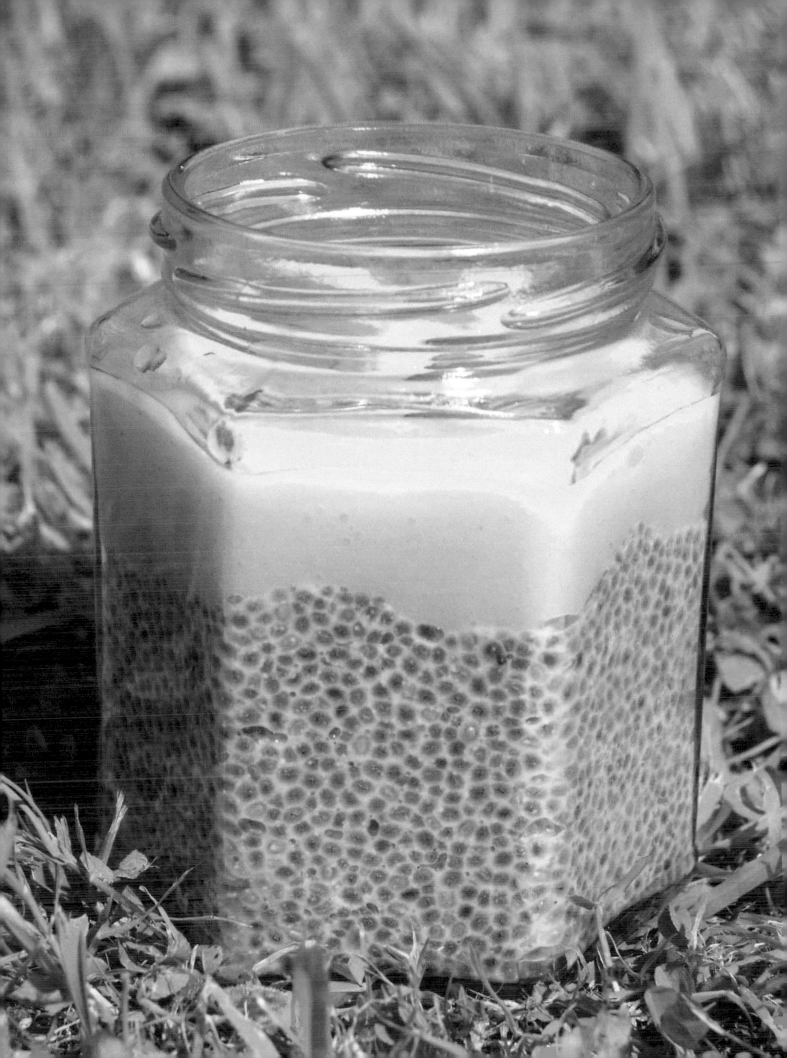

Chocolate Caramel Slice

Makes 12 slices | 10 mins (raw) (p)

Quick and easy chocolate caramel slice, aka millionaire's shortbread. It's dairy and gluten free with a fruit and nut base, a cashew caramel middle and chocolate topping. This looks impressive but can be made in less than 10 mins if you're quick.

You can use any chocolate you like for the topping. I usually use a very dark 85% cocoa solids chocolate. If you want to make your own raw chocolate topping mix together 1/3 cacao powder with 1/3 fat and 1/3 sweetener. You can use coconut oil or cacao butter for the fat.

Caramel

- 1 cup / 150g **Cashews**
- 4 tbsp **Coconut butter / oil**
- 4 tbsp **Maple syrup**, Any runny sweetener would do but you may need to adjust the quantity by taste
- 1 tsp **Vanilla**, extract or the seeds from ½ a pod

Base

- 1 cup / 150g **Figs**
- 1½ cups / 150g **Walnuts**

Topping

- 3.5oz / 100g **Chocolate**, your favourite. See intro for making a raw chocolate topping.

Equipment

- Small blender & Square tray 8"

Method

1. Blend together the walnuts and figs until they are combined into a ball.
2. Spread this out on a tray that's about 8" by 8".
3. Melt the creamed coconut / oil.
4. Add this melted coconut with all the other caramel ingredients to a blender and whizz until a smooth caramel is formed. If it becomes too thick to blend just add some hot water, 1 tbsp at a time until you can blend it smooth.
5. Melt the chocolate and spread over the top.
6. Store in the fridge and it will last for 3-4 days in theory, but mine is always eaten way before then.

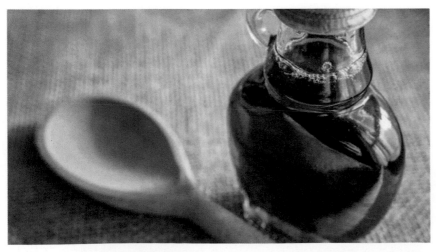

Sweeteners

In these recipes I use sweeteners that are natural like maple syrup, dates and coconut sugar. These are high in sugar but they also contain vitamins and minerals as they are not totally re-fined. Sweeteners are interchangeable in these recipes. My favourite type is homemade date syrup as it's cheap to make by blending dates and water.

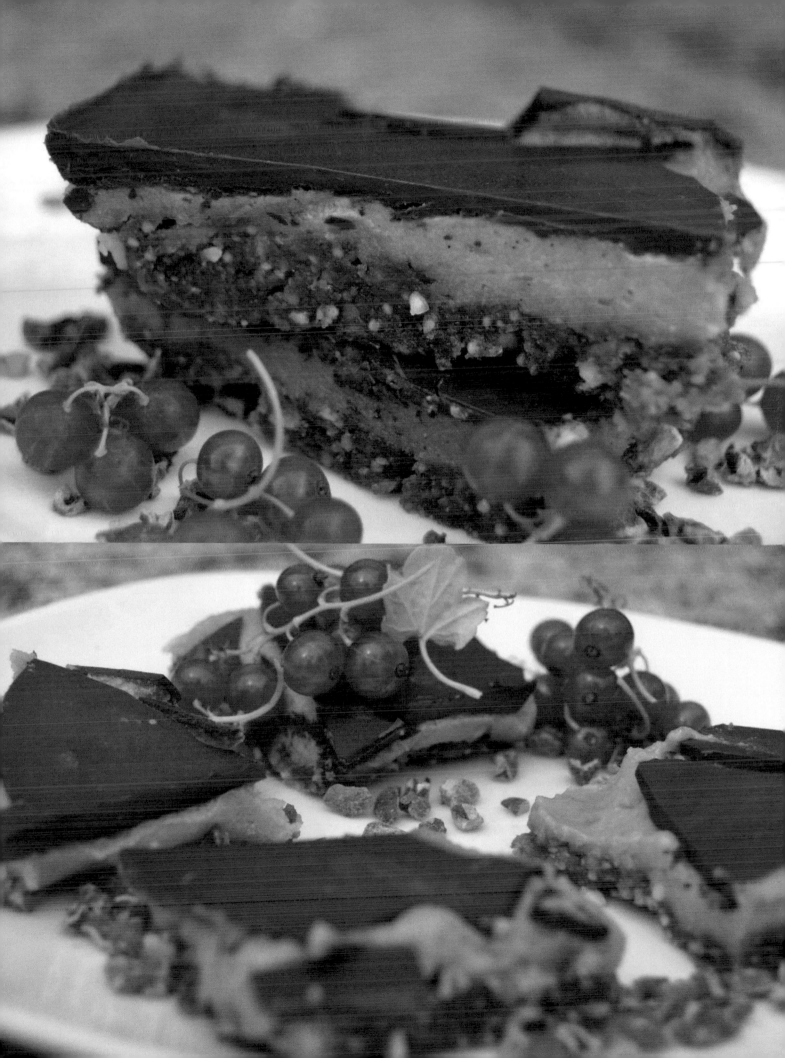

Instant Strawberry Cashew Ice Cream

Makes 4 portions | 10 mins **raw** **p**

The best things in life are simple and this instant strawberry cashew ice cream with just 4 ingredients is a perfect example. No churning or waiting is required, just a minute of blending and you will have frozen and thick ice cream.

The trick to this quick recipe is to use frozen strawberries. You can buy these pre-frozen or freeze your own, but you will need to de-stem before freezing.

Ingredients
- 1 handful **Cashews**
- ½ a handful **Dates**
- 1½ handfuls **Frozen strawberries**
- ½ tsp extract **Vanilla**, ½ a pod scraped

Equipment
- Blender

Method
1. Place the cashews, dates and vanilla in a blender and cover with water.
2. Whizz up until all is smooth.
3. Add the frozen strawberries to the blender and then blend again until they are all broken.
4. If you have a blender with a tamper you can use this to push the strawberries towards the blade.
5. You may need to add more water if it isn't mixing or more frozen strawberries if it's too runny.
6. It should be frozen enough that you can turn the blender upside down and none falls out.

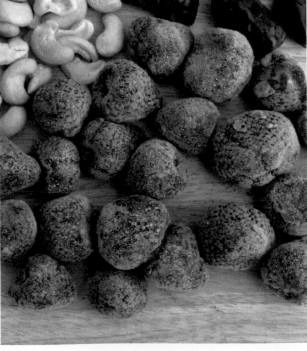

Frozen Fruit

If you don't live in a tropical climate or have spring time weather all year round then frozen fruit is a useful addition to a plant-based diet. The fruit is frozen when it's at peak ripeness and nutrition. This is particularly useful for fruit like mango where imported fresh can be very hit and miss.

Usually no chemicals are used when fruit is frozen, unlike fresh food where chemicals can be used during transportation. Frozen fruit often has just as many nutrients (sometimes more) than fresh. Several studies have concluded that frozen is nutritionally similar if not more nutritious to fresh produce. It is best to have a mix of both fresh and frozen produce for a good range of vitamins.

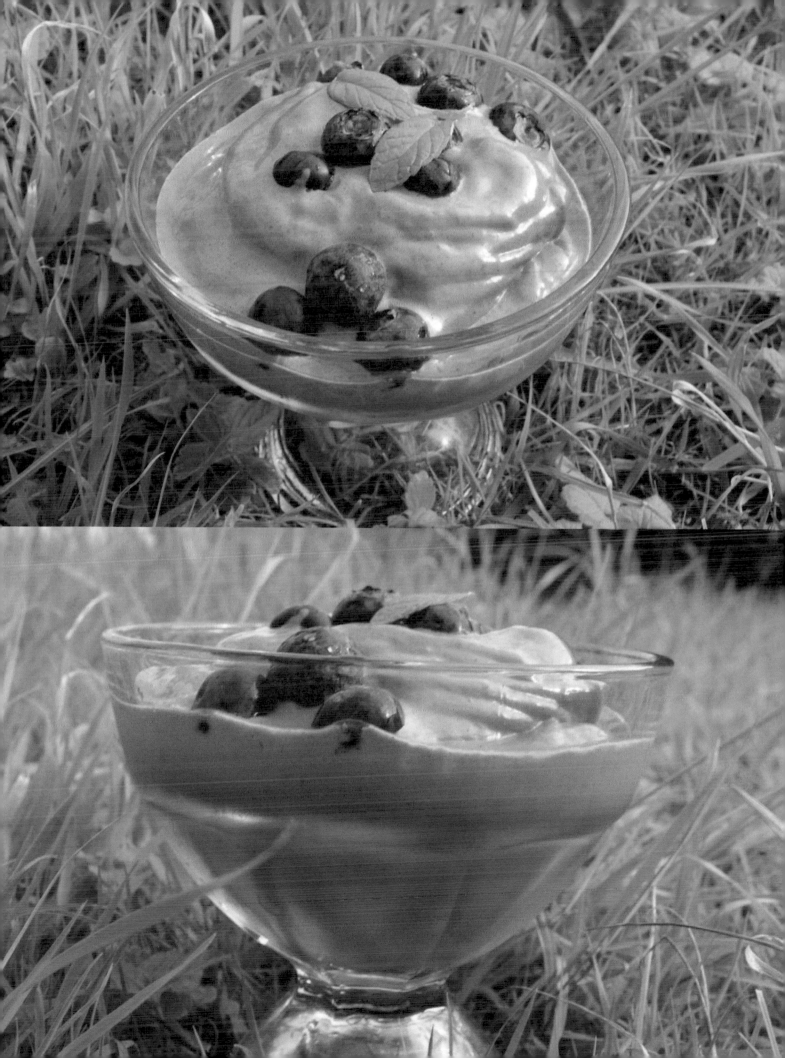

Almond Butter Strawberry Jelly Slices

Makes 16 slices | 20 mins

Creamy almond butter cut with a tangy fresh strawberry jam makes these slices incredibly moreish. The best thing about these healthy slices is you will often feel full and content after a few as they are high in fibre and made from whole unrefined ingredients.

Almond Butter Fudge Base

- 1 cup / 250g **Almond Butter**
- 1¼ cups / 120g shredded **Coconut**
- 3 tbsp **Coconut sugar,** or another sweetener like maple syrup
- 1 tsp **Vanilla**
- pinch of **Salt**, optional

Strawberry Jelly

- 2 cups / 300g **Strawberries**, halved
- 1 **Lemon**
- 2 tbsp **Sweetener**, like date / maple / coconut
- 1 tsp **Agar Agar Powder** (page 94)
- ½ cup / 120ml **Water**

Method

1. Place all the nut fudge ingredients into a food processor and blend until they are broken up and combined.
2. Spread the nut mixture onto a lined pan about 8" square and press down firmly.
3. Place all of the jelly ingredients into a pan and bring to a simmer.
4. Simmer for 5 minutes stirring constantly making the shape of 8 and 0 to make sure nothing sticks to the bottom.
5. Take the jam off the heat for 2 minutes and mash any large bits of strawberry.
6. Pour the jam on the base and chill for half an hour to set.
7. Enjoy within 3 days and keep stored in the fridge.

Notes

- You can use any nut or seed butter to make these and it will work just as well. For a nut-free diet, I recommend sunflower seed butter.

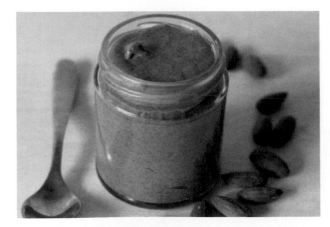

Sprouted Almond Butter

Making your own activated almond nut butter is a fun and tasty way to get the freshest nut butter around.

Soak **Almonds** overnight in **Salted Water**, drain then either dehydrate (raw) or bake at a low temperature.

Then using a food processor blend while taking breaks to scrape down the sides. This takes 10-12 minutes in a powerful food processor.

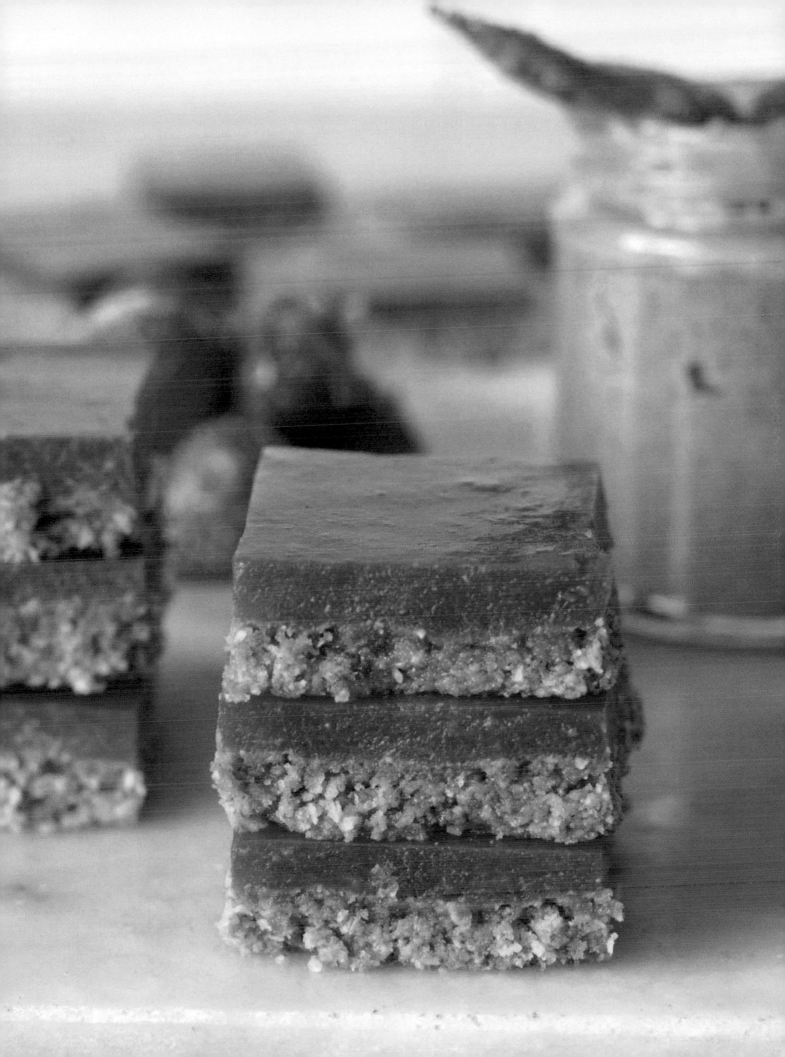

Chocolate Avocado Mousse with Salted Caramel

Serves 4 | 15 mins

This chocolate avocado mousse has a salted caramel topping and a biscuit base. It could not be simpler to make and is dairy free, gluten free and refined sugar free.

All it takes is a blending of each layer then pouring together. There is no added oil but it is creamy and decadent with the cashews and avocado. The photo below is mousse on baked sweet potato.

Base

- 1 cup / 150g **Hazelnuts**
- ½ cup / 80g **Dates**

Chocolate Avocado Mousse

- 2 **Avocados**
- 4 tbsp **Cacao powder**
- 1 cup / 240ml **Almond milk** or similar
- 1 tsp **Vanilla**
- 3-4 tbsp **Maple syrup**

Salted Caramel Topping

- 1 cup / 150g **Cashews**
- 1 cup / 175g **Dates**
- 1 tsp **Vanilla**
- 1 tsp **Sea salt** / pink salt

Equipment

- Small blender
- Glasses or jars

Method

1. Blend the base ingredients until they are all broken up and stuck together in a ball.
2. Scoop out the avocados and blend together with all the other mousse ingredients.
3. You may need to add some more milk to help the blender make a smooth mousse.
4. Taste the mousse and add more sweetener if needed. I usually use 3 tbsp but you may need to double this if you prefer a sweeter dessert.
5. Blend all of the salted caramel ingredients together with enough water to make a silky smooth caramel.
6. Push the base into the serving pot, spoon on the mousse, pour the salted caramel and then top with chopped nuts.
7. Enjoy immediately or store in the fridge and eat within 3 days.

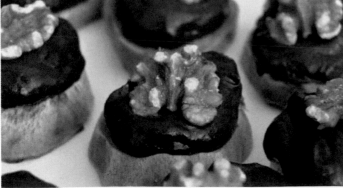

Chocolate and Avocado

Many people are put off by the idea of mixing chocolate and avocado together. However avocado has a mild taste that I don't think you can taste after mixing with rich chocolate. The avocado is just used for its creamy texture and heart healthy fats. In my experience no one can taste the avocado unless they know it's there!

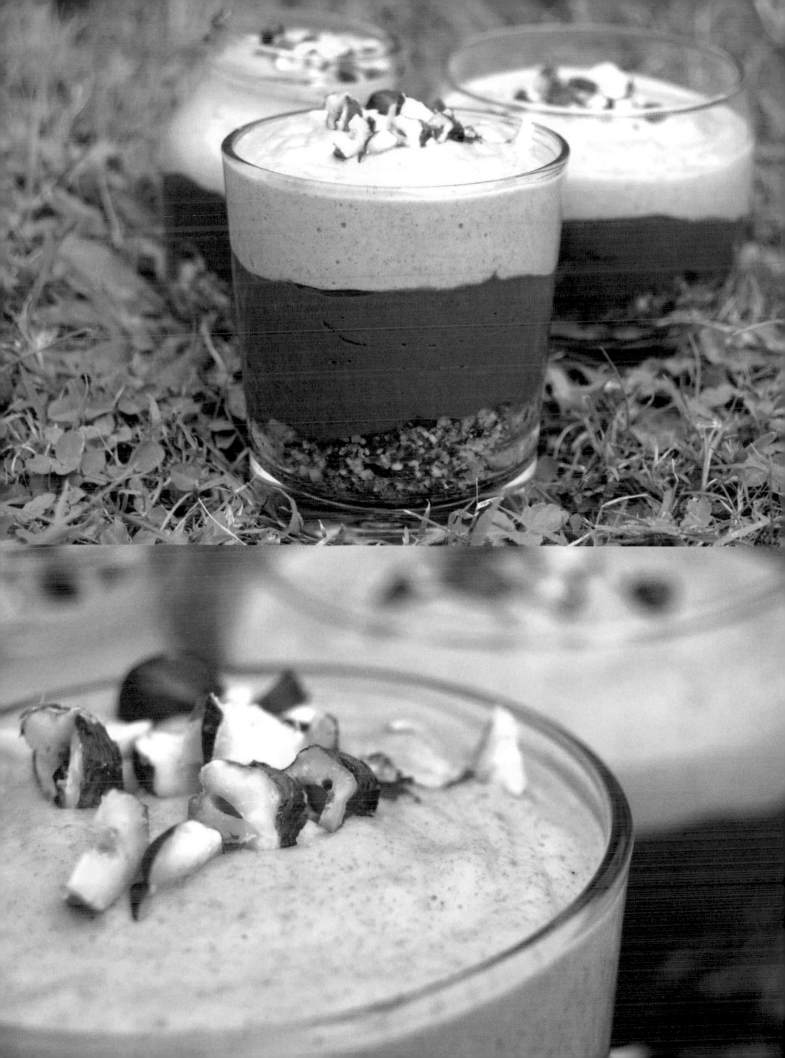

Oat Apple Crumble & Raw Custard

Makes 8 servings | 45 mins

This easy to make healthy apple crumble uses bananas and oats to give a crispy and chewy topping. No sugar is added and all the sweetness comes from fruit.

I grind gluten-free oats to make the topping but it's important to choose oats that crumble easily as they give the right texture.

Apple Crumble (nf)

- 1 cup / 175g **Dates**
- 3 large **Apples**, cooking varieties work best
- 3 **Bananas**
- 1 tsp **Vanilla**
- 1 tbsp **Cinnamon**
- 1½ cups / 150g gluten free **Oats**, finely ground
- 1 cup / 240ml **Water**

Raw Custard (raw)

- ½ cup / 75g **Cashew nuts**
- ½ cup / 80g **Dates**
- ¼ tsp **Turmeric**
- 1 tsp **Vanilla**
- 1 cup / 240ml **Water**

Equipment

- Blender / grinder for the oats
- Oven and 8" Baking dish

Method

1. Blend together the dates, vanilla and water for the crumble until smooth.
2. Core the apples and cut into small chunks, roughly 3/4 of an inch. You can peel the apples if you prefer a smooth texture. I keep the peel on, as it contains many of the nutrients.
3. Mix the apples and date paste together and put in a baking pan.
4. Grind your oats into a fine powder using a coffee grinder or small blender jug. You can use instant oats instead of grinding. The volume of 1½ cups is for whole oats.
5. Mash the bananas and mix with the ground oats and then spread on top of the apple mixture.
6. Bake at 350 F / 180 C for 35-40 minutes until the top is golden brown.
7. Blend together all of the custard ingredients until smooth. You may want to blend for a few minutes to make the custard warm or instead use warm water.
8. Serve as soon as the apple crumble comes out of the oven. Keep leftovers in the fridge where they will last a few days.

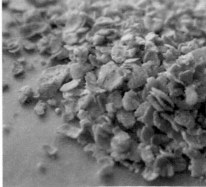

Oats and Gluten

This recipe book is gluten-free but several recipes do use oats. Oats are naturally gluten-free but many do contain gluten due to contamination. They can be contaminated by wheat and other grains during the factory processing or when they are grown. Use gluten-free oats if you have a gluten sensitivity. These are suitable for most gluten intolerant people. Some may also be intolerant to GF oats as they contain avenin and this is similar to gluten.

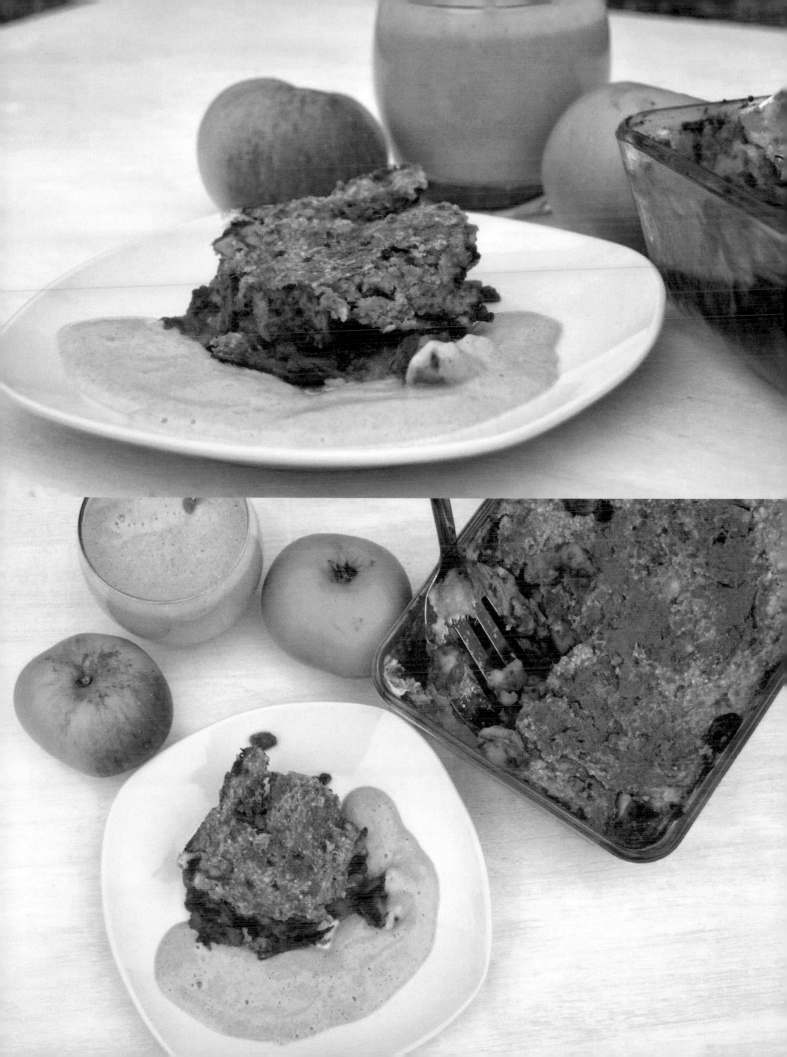

Coco Cacao Chocolate Spread

Makes 8 servings | 5 mins **p** **nf**

This Coco Cacao Chocolate Spread could not be easier to make – just blend together the ingredients, chill and enjoy. I've added vanilla to give some extra depth but it's also great without.

Ingredients

- 1 can **Coconut milk**, not low-fat 15oz / 400ml
- 4 tbsp **Cacao/Cocoa powder**
- 4 tbsp **Coconut sugar**
- 1 tsp **Vanilla**

Equipment

- Blender

Method

1. Place everything in a blender and blend for 1-2 minutes until everything is mixed.
2. Chill for a few hours in the fridge and it's ready.
3. Keep in the fridge and use within a week.

Notes

Use coconut milk without additives and stabilisers. The additives keep the milk as a liquid and you want the type of coconut milk that separates into cream and water. Check your coconut milk is suitable by shaking and ensuring the fat and water are somewhat separated.

Chocolate pudding and Chocolate Ice Pops

This recipe can also be used to make:

- **Chocolate mousse puddings**, pour into small dishes, then chill and top with grated chocolate.

- **Chocolate ice pops**, pour the mixture into pop moulds then freeze.

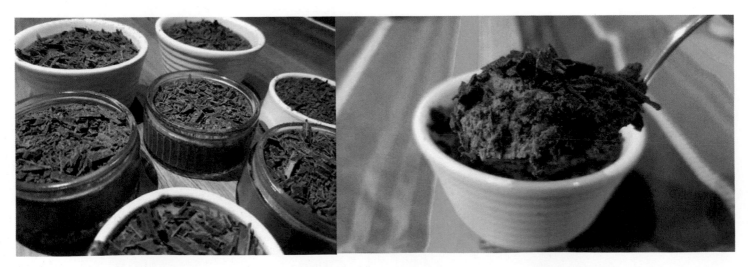

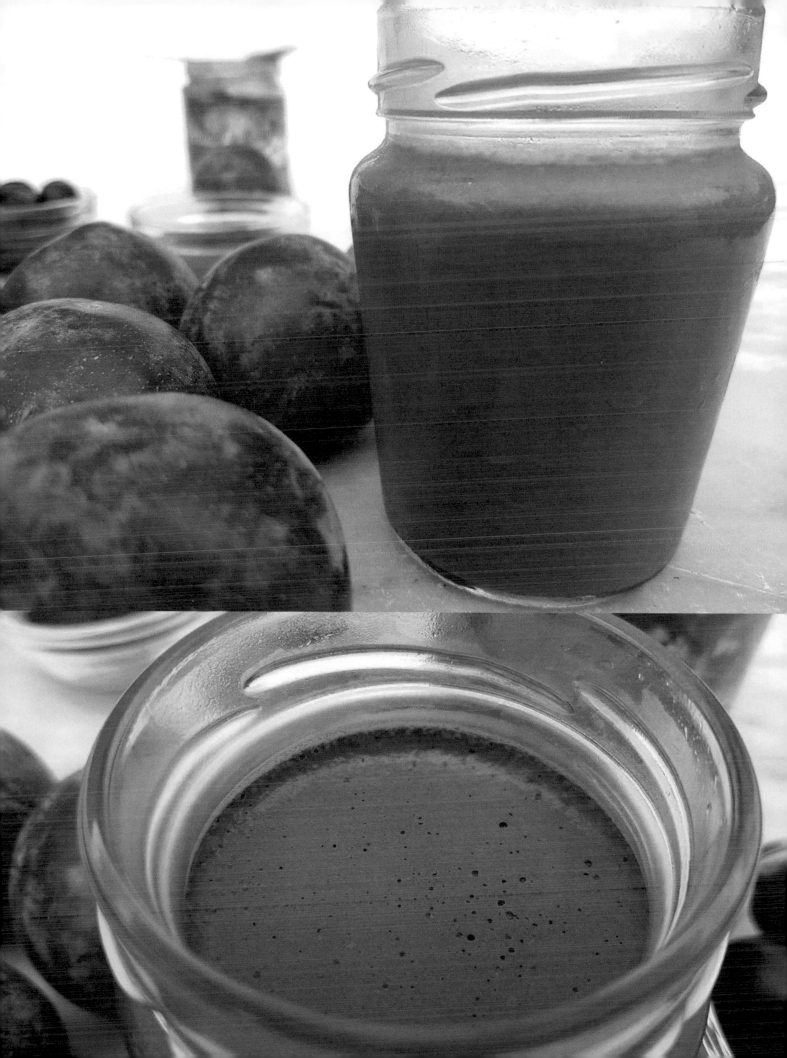

Chocolate Sunflower Kale Crisps

Makes 8 servings | 40 mins baked | 10.5h raw (raw) (p) (nf)

Dates and Cacao make these sweet kale crisps very moreish. Even people that are not fans of kale love these crisps as the kale is just a crispy and almost unrecognisable base.

Ingredients

- 1 cup / 140g **Sunflower seeds**
- 14oz / 400g **Kale**, still on stems
- 8-12 **Dates**, pitted
- 4 tbsp **Cocoa/Cacao powder**
- 1 tsp **Vanilla**
- pinch of **Salt**
- ½ cup / 120ml **Water**
- **Water** and pinch of **Salt** for soaking

Equipment

- Blender
- Oven/Dehydrator
- Greaseproof paper

Method

1. Soak the sunflower seeds in water with a pinch of salt. Overnight is best.
2. Rip the kale off the stems. Remove up to where the stem snaps.
3. Place the kale in a bowl and sprinkle over a pinch of salt.
4. Scrunch the kale up using your hands until it's halved in size.
5. Drain the sunflower seeds and place with all the other ingredients into a blender then blend until smooth.
6. Pour the sunflower sauce onto the kale and massage to coat all the leaves.
7. Baked or Raw:
   - **Bake**; spread out thinly onto a lined tray and bake at 300F / 150C for about 25-30 minutes. Toss every 5-10 minutes and take out of the oven as soon as they are dry. Watch like a hawk as they burn easily.
   - **Raw**; spread out thinly onto a non-stick sheet. Dry at 110F / 43C for 10-12 hours tossing half way.
8. Enjoy the kale crisps straight after cooking / drying.
9. Once cooled they can be stored in an airtight container for a few weeks, but it's best to have them the same day as they lose their crispiness.

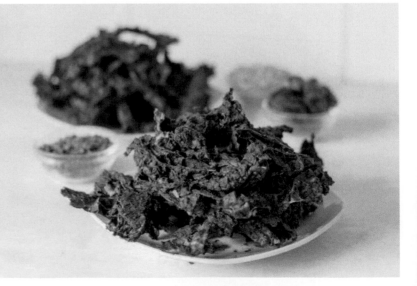

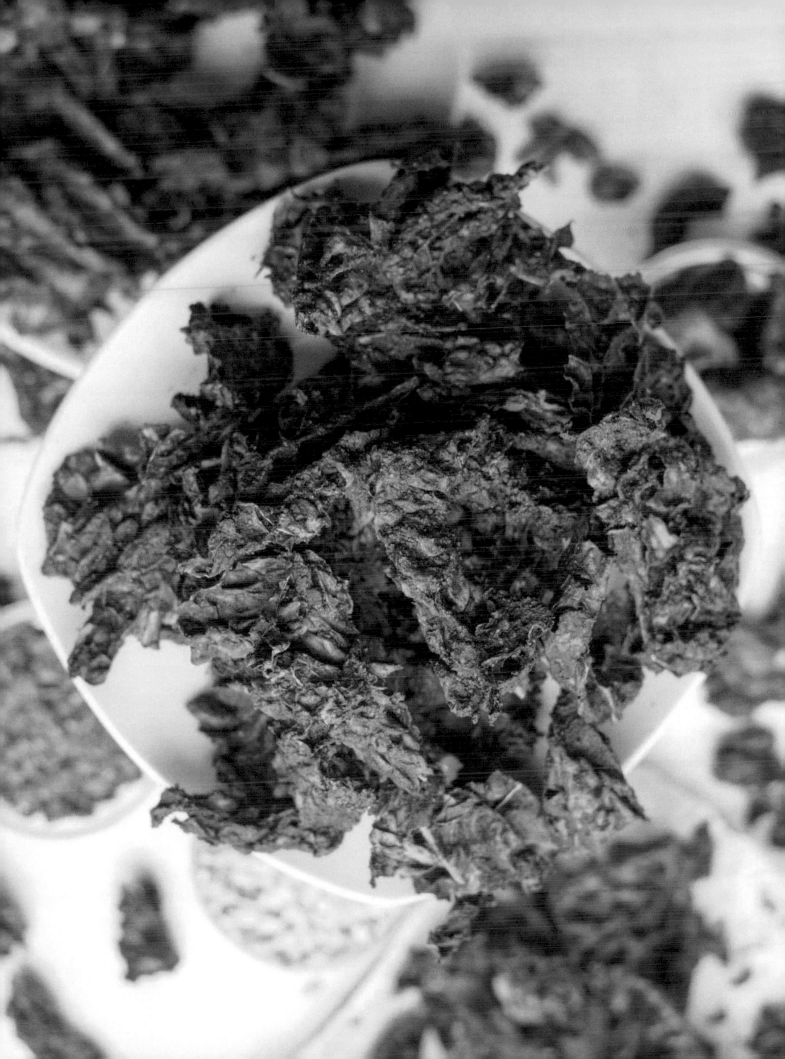

Raspberry Chocolate Doughnut Peaches

Makes 5 doughnuts | 30 mins

Doughnut peaches / Saturn peaches / flat peaches / paraguayas - whatever you call them, they are only in season for a short amount of time so make the most when they are! This recipe for healthy raspberry chocolate doughnut peaches is easy and fun. The peaches have a chocolate shell and a thick layer of raspberry cashew cream.

Ingredients

- 5 **Doughnut peaches**, de-stoned and peeled
- 1 cup / 125g **Raspberries**
- 1 cup / 150g **Cashew nuts**
- 2-3 tbsp **Date syrup**, or any sweetener
- 1 tsp **Vanilla**
- 2 tbsp **Coconut oil / butter**
- 4.4oz / 125g **Chocolate,** use raw for raw

Toppings

- **Fruit** and **nuts**, such as raspberries, blueberries, pistachios and hazelnuts

Equipment

- Small blender / food processor
- Double boiler
- Non-stick sheet

Method

1. Push out the stone and peel all of the peaches, making sure not to break the fruit.
2. Put peaches in the freezer for about 30 minutes.
3. Push the raspberries through a sieve using a wooden spoon and collect all the raspberry juice.
4. Melt the coconut oil / cream.
5. Blend together the raspberry juice, cashews, date syrup, vanilla and melted coconut until smooth.
6. Pour the raspberry cream into a bowl and cover each peach with it. Then place on a non stick sheet in the freezer for 30 minutes.
7. Melt the chocolate then spoon it over each peach until they are covered. Sprinkle with fruit or nuts on top. Put back on non stick sheet in the fridge.
8. Enjoy immediately or store in the fridge where they will last a couple of days.

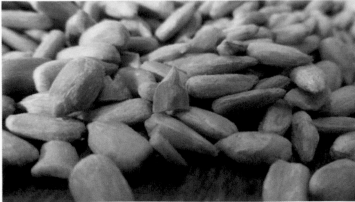

Nut Free Adaptation - use sunflower seeds

I often use sunflower seeds in place of most nuts in recipes. It won't quite have the same flavour but will give a very similar texture.

Also it makes the dish more affordable as sunflower seeds are a fraction the cost of many nuts.

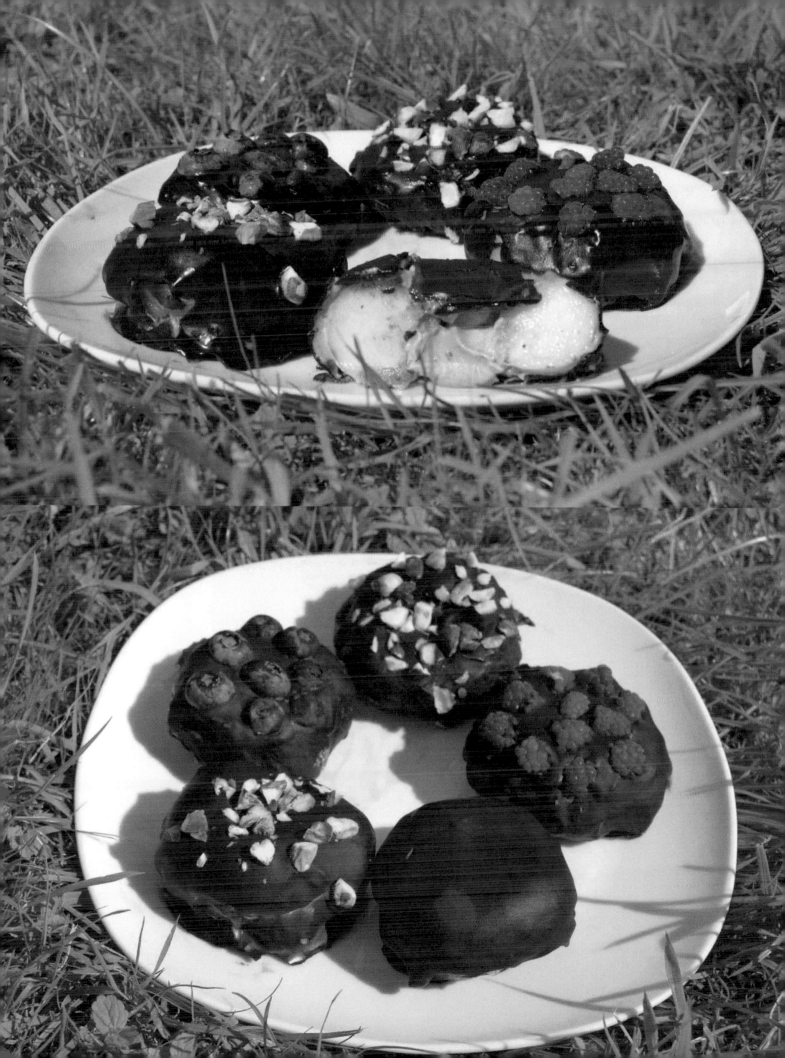

Fruit and Seed Chocolate Rice Cakes

Makes 12 rice cakes | 20 mins **nf**

These Dark Chocolate covered Rice Cakes with fruit and seeds taste even better than they look! The perfect mixture of crunchy seeds, chewy fruit, crispy brown rice cakes and rich dark chocolate make for a delicious healthy snack. What can be a better way to eat a rainbow of different foods to ensure you get a range of vitamins and minerals from natural produce?

Ingredients

- 4.4oz / 125g **Dark Chocolate**
- 12 **Brown rice cakes**
- 2 tbsp **Sunflower Seeds**
- 2 tbsp **Raisins**
- 2 tbsp **Pumpkin Seeds**
- 2 tbsp **Goji Berries**
- 2 tbsp **Cacao Nibs**
- 2 tbsp **Mulberries**
- 2 tbsp **Shredded coconut**
- 2 tbsp **Sesame seeds**

Equipment

- Double boiler

Notes

I've made these very successfully in a hotel without a kitchen. You can melt the chocolate in a mug surrounded by hot water in the sink. Then spoon and spread the chocolate with a teaspoon before sprinkling with seeds and fruit.

Method

1. Chop the chocolate up and melt 3/4 in a bowl over hot water. Pick a bowl with a flat area that's at least the size of a rice cake.
2. Add the last 1/4 of the chocolate and stir off the heat until melted for easy tempering.
3. Dip the rice cake in the chocolate to coat then sprinkle with the toppings.
4. Place in the fridge for 10 minutes to set and enjoy.
5. Store in an airtight container once set as they will go soft otherwise. Best eaten on the day made.

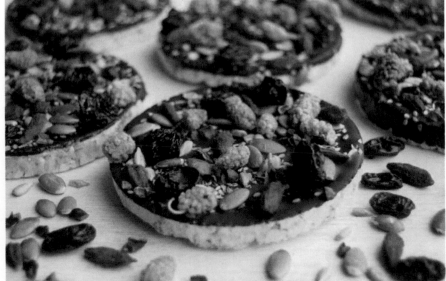

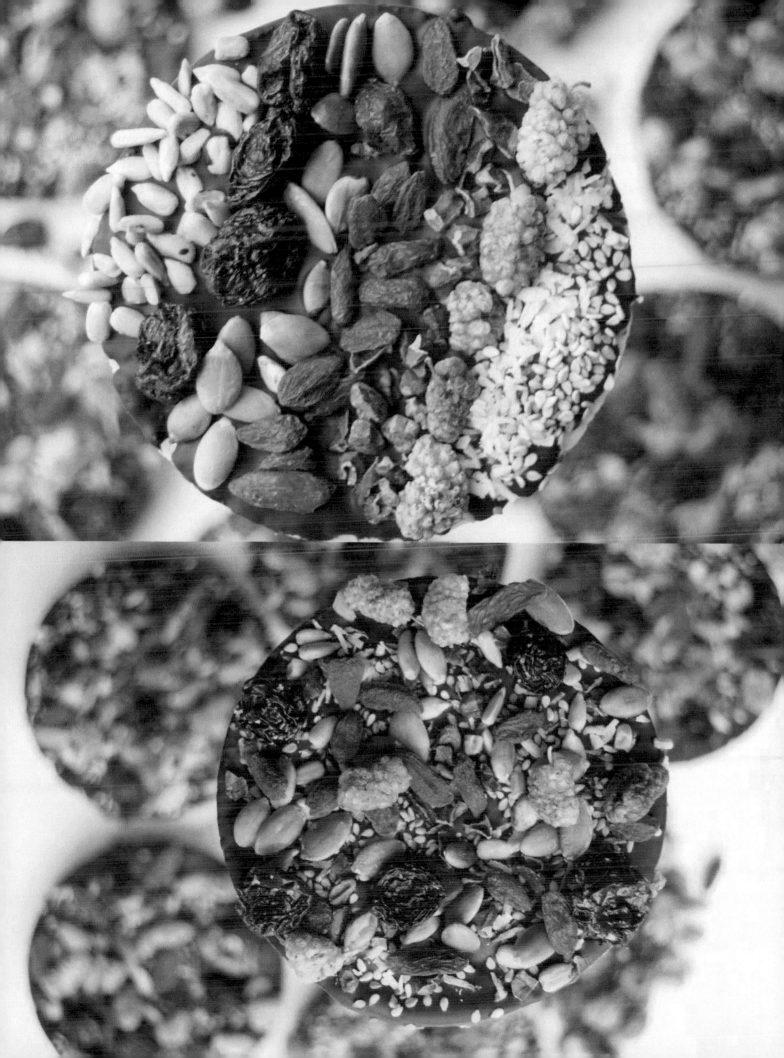

Coconut Almond Ice-Cream

Serves 4 | 20 mins 🅟

Easy to make dairy-free and healthy chocolate ice-cream without a machine. The best compliment I've had with this ice cream is that is tastes like normal (premium high-end) chocolate ice cream. The simple recipes are often the best.

Ingredients

- 1 Can full fat **Coconut Milk,** 14oz / 400ml
- 3 tbsp **Cacao / Cocoa powder**
- 3 tbsp **Coconut sugar**
- 2 tbsp **Ground almonds**
- 1 tsp **Vanilla**

Equipment

- Electric whisk
- Bowl
- Dish 8" square

Method

1. Empty the coconut milk into a bowl, using all the cream and the water.
2. Whisk for 2-3 minutes with an electric whisk on high to incorporate as much air as possible. You can use a manual whisk but it will be quite time-consuming, about 10 minutes and a good workout.
3. Add all the other ingredients and then whisk on low to incorporate. Scrape down the sides to ensure it's all mixed.
4. Test the mixture and adjust sweetness/bitterness to taste. I like it quite bitter so usually add less sweetener.
5. Pour into a dish then freeze for 3-4 hours.
6. Remove from the freezer when it's frozen, I use a toothpick to check this.
7. Leave to stand for 5 minutes at room temp before serving.
8. It will last several weeks in the freezer but will need to deforest a bit first and have a good stir if left in for longer than the 3-4 hours.

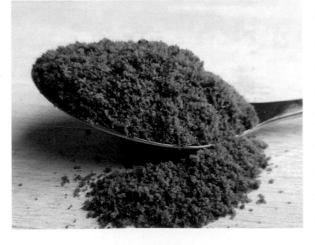

Coconut Sugar

Coconut sugar is made by collecting the sap of the coconut flower buds and evaporating until solid sugar crystals are formed.

It contains several vitamins including iron, zinc, calcium and potassium.

Coconut sugar is still a sugar so should be consumed in moderation (just like dates and maple) but does have several advantages over normal refined sugar.

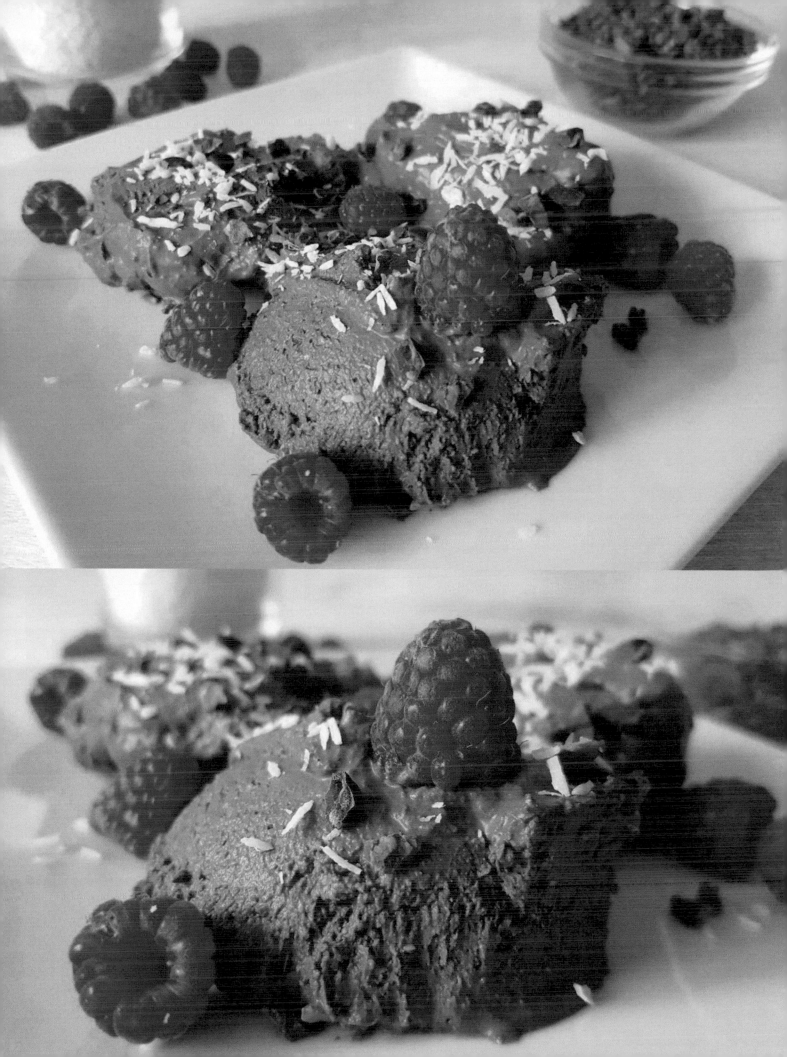

Chocolate Protein Mousse

Serves 4 | 20 mins **nf**

This easy to make creamy and velvety mousse is made from just a tin of white beans and very dark chocolate.

Both beans and dark chocolate are high in protein. Dark chocolate has a high cocoa content from the ground cocoa beans. One serving contains about 9g of protein and also a healthy amount of iron, manganese and calcium.

Ingredients

- 1 tin **White / Cannellini beans**, 15oz / 400ml
- 150g **Dark Chocolate**

Equipment

- Blender and Electric whisk
- Sieve and Bowl

Method

1. Melt most of the chocolate in a bowl over hot water.
2. Leave enough chocolate to grate for a topping.
3. Pour the beans into a sieve with a bowl below to catch all the bean juice.
4. Whisk the bean juice with an electric whisk for a few minutes while the chocolate melts.
5. Add the beans to the melted chocolate and blend together in a jug blender or food processor. You may have to scrape down the sides several times.
6. Continue to whisk the bean juice (aka aquafaba) until stiff peaks are formed, this takes about 8-10 minutes in total with an electric whisk.
7. Stiff peaks are when you can turn the bowl upside down and the mixture doesn't move, see the photo below. With aquafaba you don't need to worry about over-whisking.
8. Fold the chocolate bean mixture into the aquafaba then pour into 4 dishes.
9. Chill for an hour then sprinkle with grated chocolate.
10. Keep in the fridge and enjoy within 3 days.

Two Ingredient Chocolate Mousse

You can make a two ingredient mousse just by folding in the melted chocolate into the whipped bean juice. This makes a lighter mousse with significantly less carbohydrates and protein.

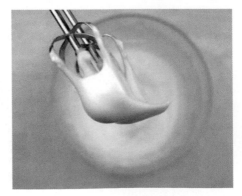

Aquafaba

This is the name of the liquid made when beans and other legumes are cooked in water. It was named after the Latin for water (aqua) and bean (faba). It's most common application is to make vegan meringues but has many uses due to its emulsifying and thickening properties. You can either use the bean juice from a can or from beans you've cooked from dry.

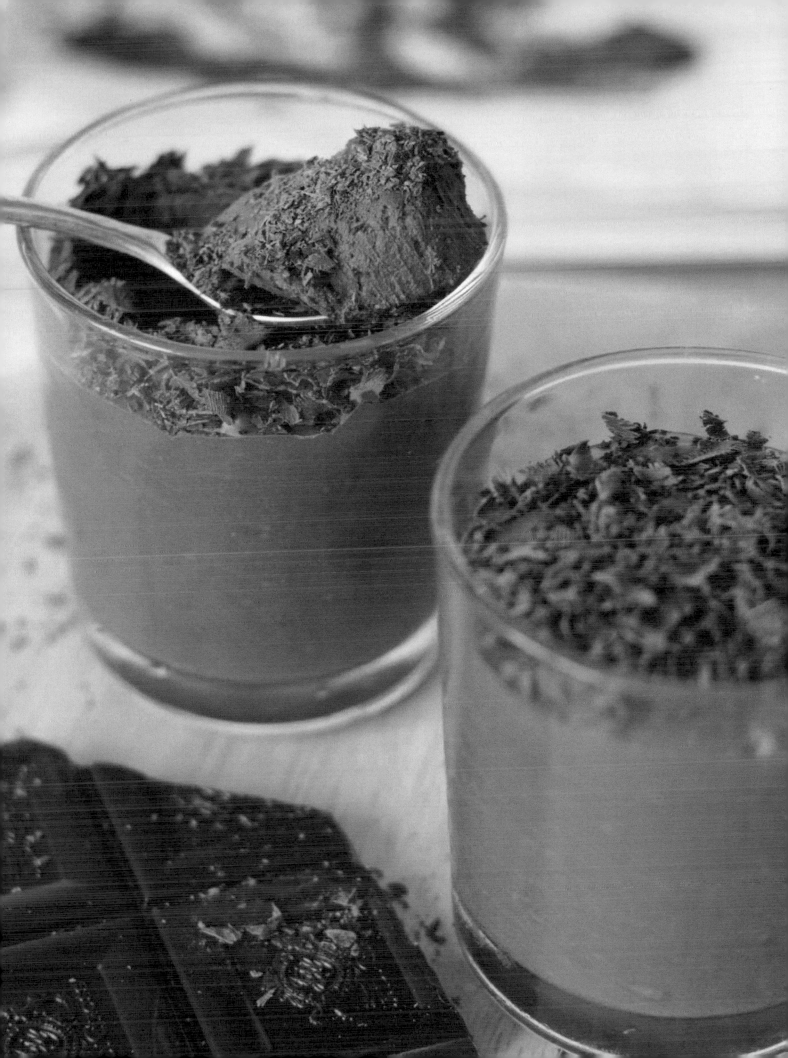

Smoked Cashew Cheese

Makes 12 servings | 15 mins

This smoked cashew vegan cheese is sweet, creamy and very moreish. Full of heart-healthy fats, vitamins and protein. The cheesy dairy free taste comes from nutritional yeast and the smokiness is provided by smoked paprika. It's quick and easy to make as it isn't fermented.

Ingredients

- 1 cup / 150g **Cashews**
- ½ cup / 40g **Nutritional Yeast** (page 108)
- 1 tbsp **Smoked paprika**
- 1 tbsp **Maple syrup**
- 1 tbsp **Agar agar powder**
- 1 clove of **Garlic**
- 1 **Lemon** juiced
- ¼ tsp **Turmeric**
- ¼ tsp **Cayenne pepper**
- 1½ cups / 350ml **Water**
- pinch of **Salt**

Equipment

- Blender
- Pan
- Mould and Greaseproof paper

Smoked Paprika

The smoked flavour comes from the smoked paprika spice. It's traditionally made by drying paprika chillies over wood fires. It has a smoky and woody taste and is one of my most used spices. Remember to buy a paprika that is smoked as the sweet/hot varieties are not the same.

Method

1. Place half the water and everything else apart from the agar agar into a blender.
2. Blend until smooth.
3. In a pan put in the remaining half of the water and the agar agar.
4. Simmer for 5 minutes stirring constantly. Make sure no lumps of agar agar form at the bottom.
5. Take off the heat and stir in the cashew mixture until combined.
6. Pour into a mould lined with greaseproof paper and then chill for 2 hours.
7. Enjoy within 3 days and keep chilled.

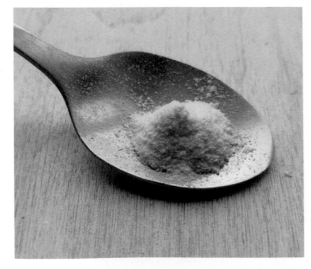

Agar Agar Powder

This is a natural seaweed extract that is a very useful gelling agent. Agar is the Malay name for the red algae that it's made from.

It can be used to set most things and just needs a short simmer to activate.

All recipes in this book use pure agar agar powder as it's the most potent form. It is available in flakes and bars but if you use these, more is needed. It can be picked up inexpensively in Asian shops.

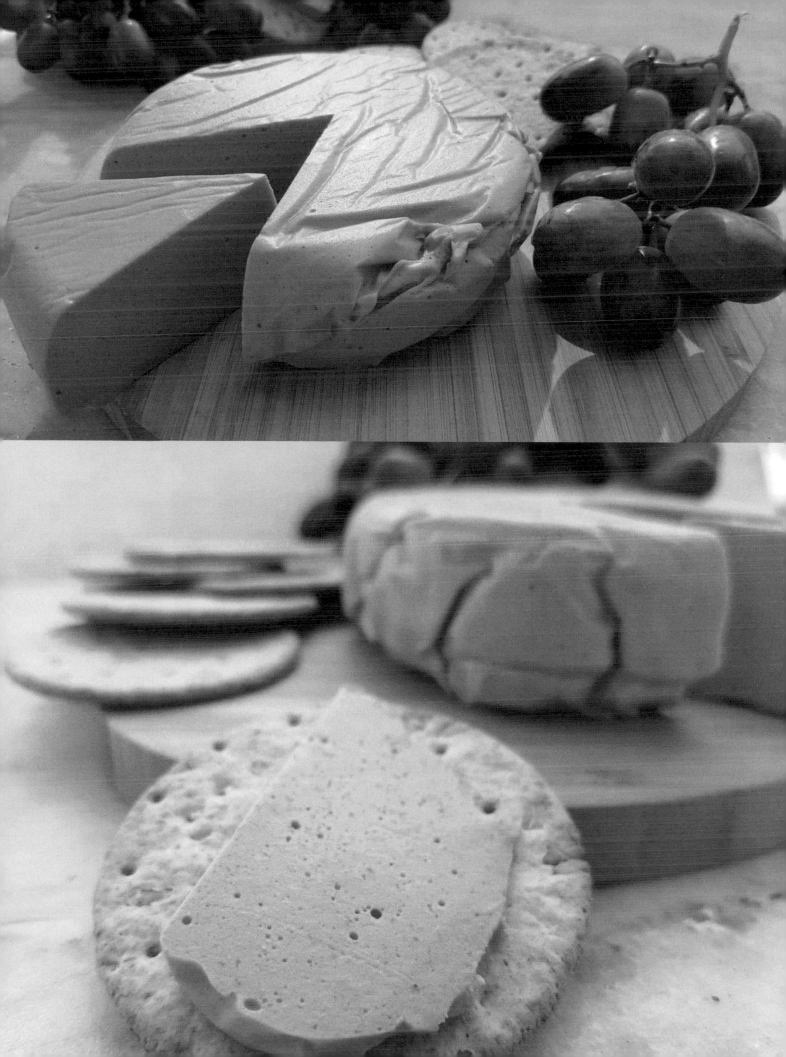

Light Queso Cheese Dip

Makes one medium bowl | 1h 15 mins (p)

This light vegan queso cheese dip contains aubergine and butternut squash to make it light and low calorie. Perfect for those days where you want something filling and creamy but not too heavy. Also great because it's high in fibre and vitamins.

Simple to make but does take some time while the veggies bake, however the oven is doing all the work while you sit back.

Ingredients

- 2 **Aubergines**
- ½ **Butternut squash**
- 1 **Onion**
- 1 clove of **Garlic**
- 2 tbsp **Cashews**
- 1 tsp **Cumin**
- ½ tsp **Cayenne pepper**
- ½ tsp **Turmeric**
- ½ cup / 40g **Nutritional Yeast** (page 108)
- 1 tsp **Salt**
- 1 tsp **Corn** or **Tapioca (P) starch**
- 2 cups / 500ml Water

Toppings

- Smoked paprika
- Chilli slices
- Chopped tomatoes

Equipment

- Blender
- Oven
- Lined roasting pan

Method

1. Cut the butternut, onion and aubergines in half and place on a baking tray.
2. Bake at 425F / 220C for about 30-45 minutes. Often you will need to take out the aubergine and onion first as the butternut takes about 15 minutes more to bake.
3. Scoop out the flesh of the butternut and aubergine, once cool. The skins are tasty to eat but they are not needed for this recipe as the dip is velvety smooth.
4. Place everything in a high-speed blender and blend for a few minutes until all broken up. You may have to blend in two batches in a small jug blender.
5. Serve the dip with smoked paprika, chopped tomatoes, chilli spices and coriander.
6. Best eaten just after made and still warm.

Serving Suggestion

In the photo I'm serving these with thick slices of baked potatoes with no oil added. This dip works really well with just about anything dippable like "Five Seed Oatcakes" on page 134 or "Tomato and Basil Lentil Chips" on page 120.

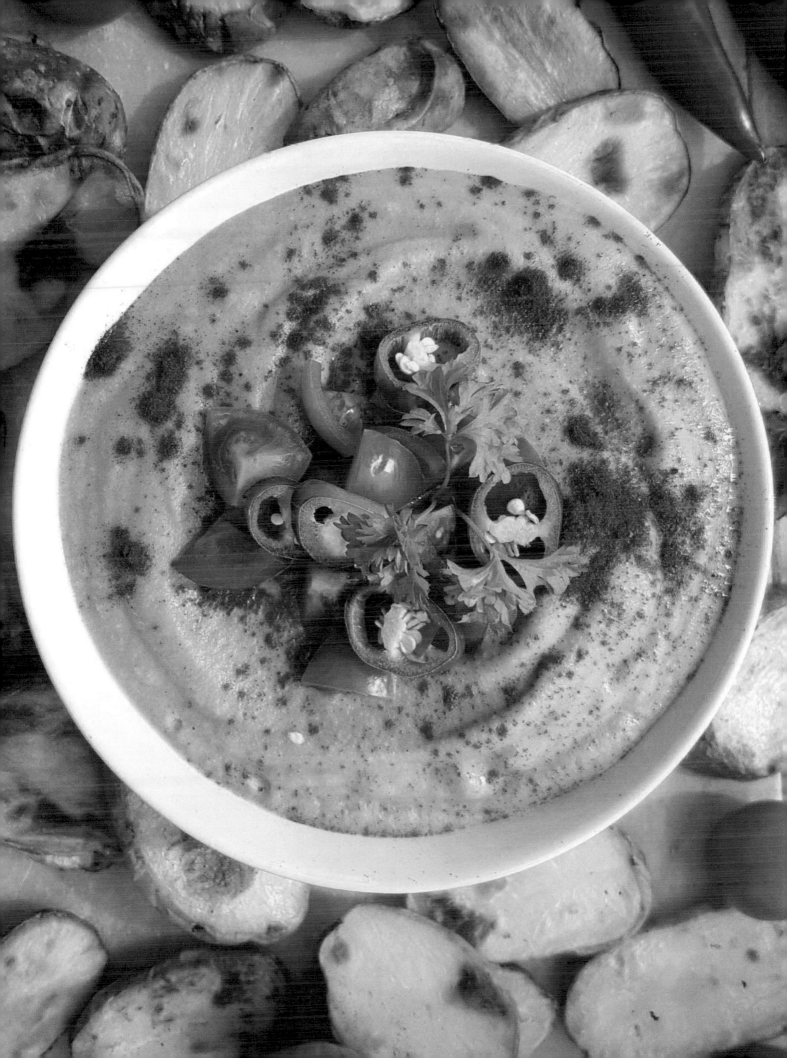

Spicy Kidney Bean Tomato Dip

Makes one medium bowl | 15 mins **nf**

A Spicy Kidney Bean Tomato Dip that is cheap, nutritious and takes a few minutes to make. This dip is a staple in my diet as I always have all the ingredients on hand and it's very budget friendly. Serve with some oatcakes or carrot sticks for a filling meal or pop in a tub to have a healthy snack on the go.

Ingredients

- 1 can **Kidney beans**, drained and rinsed
- 1 **Onion**, finely sliced
- 2 cloves of **Garlic**, peeled and diced
- a splash of **Water**, for oil free "frying"
- 4 tbsp **Tomato purée**
- ¼ tsp **Cayenne pepper**
- ¼ tsp **Turmeric**
- ¼ tsp **Cumin**
- ½ tsp **Garam masala**
- **Salt** and **pepper**, to taste
- 1 tbsp **Chia seeds**
- 1 **Lime**, juiced
- ¼ cup / 60ml **Water**

Equipment

- Pan
- Potato masher

Method

1. Add the onion, garlic and water to a pan and simmer for 4-5 minutes until softened.
2. Then add everything apart from the lime and chia and simmer for 2-3 minutes.
3. Mash the dip with a potato masher, just roughly to get a chunky but spreadable consistency.
4. Add the lime juice, chia seeds then stir and serve.
5. Tastes great either still warm or chilled from the fridge.

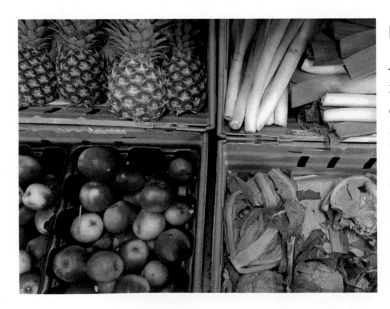

Everyday Food

After reading this book you would be forgiven for thinking that my diet mainly consists of cakes and candy.

It actually consists mainly of dishes like this that are cheap, quick and full of nutrition. Cakes are usually made once a week.

However these dishes are not particularly popular, maybe because they are too basic or well known? So I usually create more unique and interesting recipes.

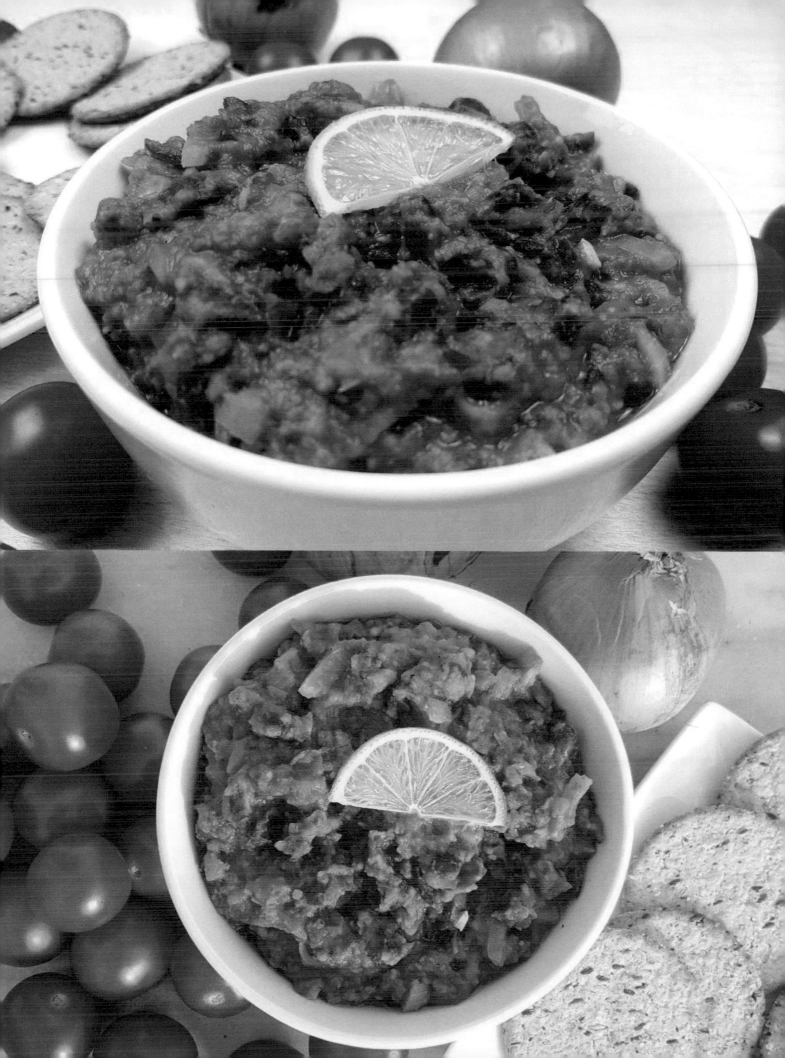

Sprouted Sunflower Cheese

Makes 6" cheese | 25 mins **p** **nf**

It slices, grates and melts so you can use it in place of regular cheese in many recipes. Heart-healthy cheese that tastes great, is cheap to make and doesn't take long – what isn't there to love about this recipe? It's one of my staples and I often have a batch in the fridge.

Ingredients

- 1 cup / 140g **Sunflower seeds**
- 1 **Lime**, juiced
- 3 tbsp **Nutritional Yeast** (page 108)
- 1 clove **Garlic**
- 1 slice of **Onion**
- ½ tsp **Turmeric**
- ¼ tsp **Cayenne pepper**
- 1 tbsp **Agar Agar Powder** (page 94)
- 1½ cups / 360ml **Water**
- 2 tbsp **Miso**, sweet white is best any is good. Replace with a pinch of salt for paleo

Equipment

- Pan, Blender and 6" dish

Method

1. Soak the sunflower seeds in water for at least 10 minutes, overnight is best.
2. In a pan mix together the agar agar with a dash of water until dissolved. Then stir in 1 cup / 240ml of water.
3. Bring the agar agar mixture to a boil and simmer for 5 minutes stirring constantly to prevent any sticking at the bottom.
4. Take the pan off the heat and allow to cool for 5 minutes.
5. Drain and rinse the sunflower seeds.
6. Place everything in a blender, apart from the agar agar mixture, with half a cup / 120 ml of water and blend until smooth.
7. Whisk together the sunflower seed mixture and the agar agar until it's all combined.
8. Pour into a dish, about 6" in diameter, and then place in the fridge for an hour to set.
9. You may want to oil your dish, but I tend to use a shiny ceramic dish and the cheese comes out easy enough without any oil.
10. Take out of the dish once set and enjoy this vegan cheese in place of normal cheese. It will last a few days in the fridge.

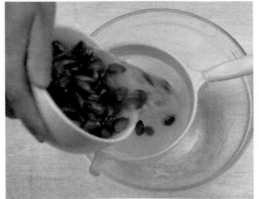

Sprouting Nuts and Seeds

This is the process of soaking nuts and seeds in salted water to start the germination. It makes the nuts / seeds easier to digest and increases the bioavailability of nutrients. Some seeds will start to open up when they are sprouted but many nuts won't. This process is also called activating.

If you're not convinced that soaking nuts or seeds is important, just look at the brown murky water when you do soak!

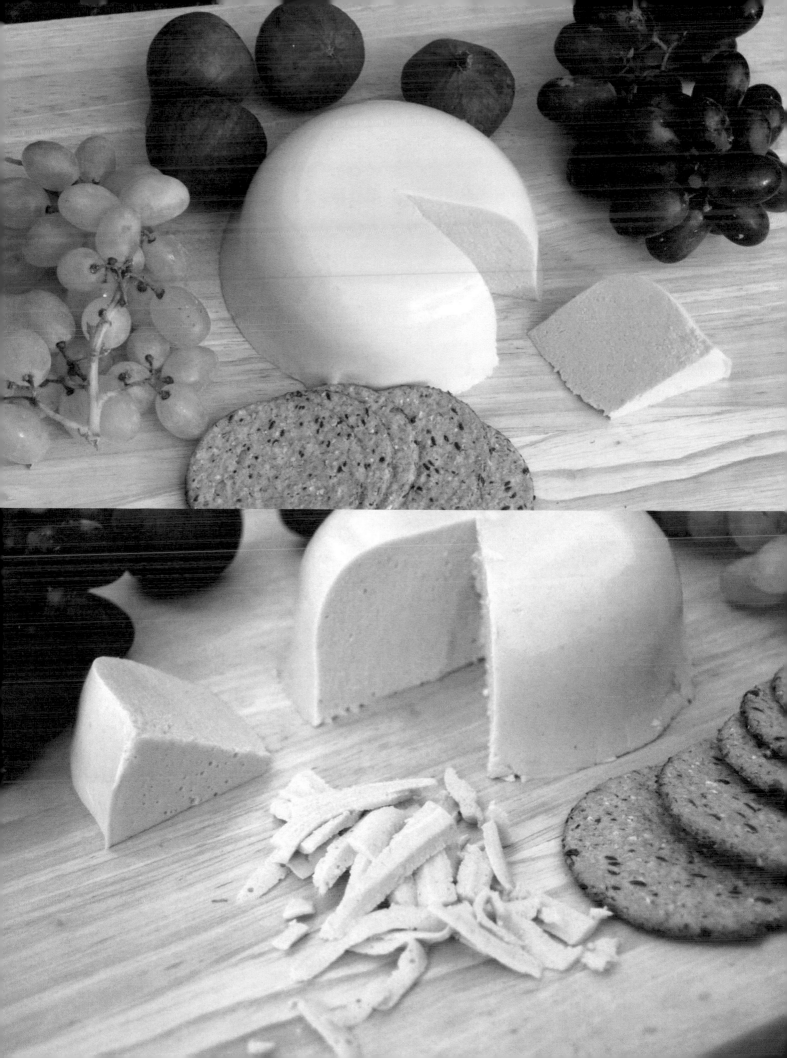

French Onion Miso Soup

Makes 4 servings | 1h 20 mins **nf**

Easy and tasty vegan French onion soup recipe that uses miso. I love French onion soup and I love miso soup and this hybrid of them is delicious but simple and easy to make. It has a rich depth of flavour but is only made from three ingredients.

Ingredients

- 6 medium **Onions**, about 2.2lb / 1kg
- 2 tbsp dark **Miso**
- 2 tbsp **Balsamic vinegar**
- 2 cups / 500ml **Water**

Optional to top

- **Oatcakes**
- **Sunflower seed cheese**, grated

Equipment

- Pan with lid

Method

1. Cut all the onions into thin slices.
2. Place in a pan, cover with a lid and cook on a very low heat for an hour. Stir every 10-15 minutes.
3. After an hour the onions should be caramelised. If not return to the heat for 10 minute intervals until they are a light brown.
4. Stir in the water, miso and balsamic vinegar. It should be warm enough to eat straight away, if not return to the heat and gently heat for a few minutes. Heating destroys much of the goodness in the miso so don't bring to a boil.
5. Serve with a slice of bread / oat cake covered in Sprouted Sunflower Cheese (page 100).
6. Any left overs will last for a few days in the fridge.

Notes

This doesn't use a huge amount of energy as the hob is set on a very low setting for the hour long cooking. On my induction cooker I usually set it to 60C.

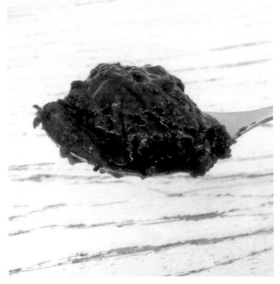

Miso

This paste is a useful ingredient in many dishes to give a salty and umami taste. There are countless different varieties with different flavours such as sweet and fruity.

It's made by fermenting beans with salt and a culture. Rice or barley is often added. The fermenting process takes 6-12 months so it's not something many people make at home.

Miso is usually made from soy beans but it is possible to make from other beans/legumes such as chickpeas.

Make sure you buy a gluten-free version if you have a reaction to gluten.

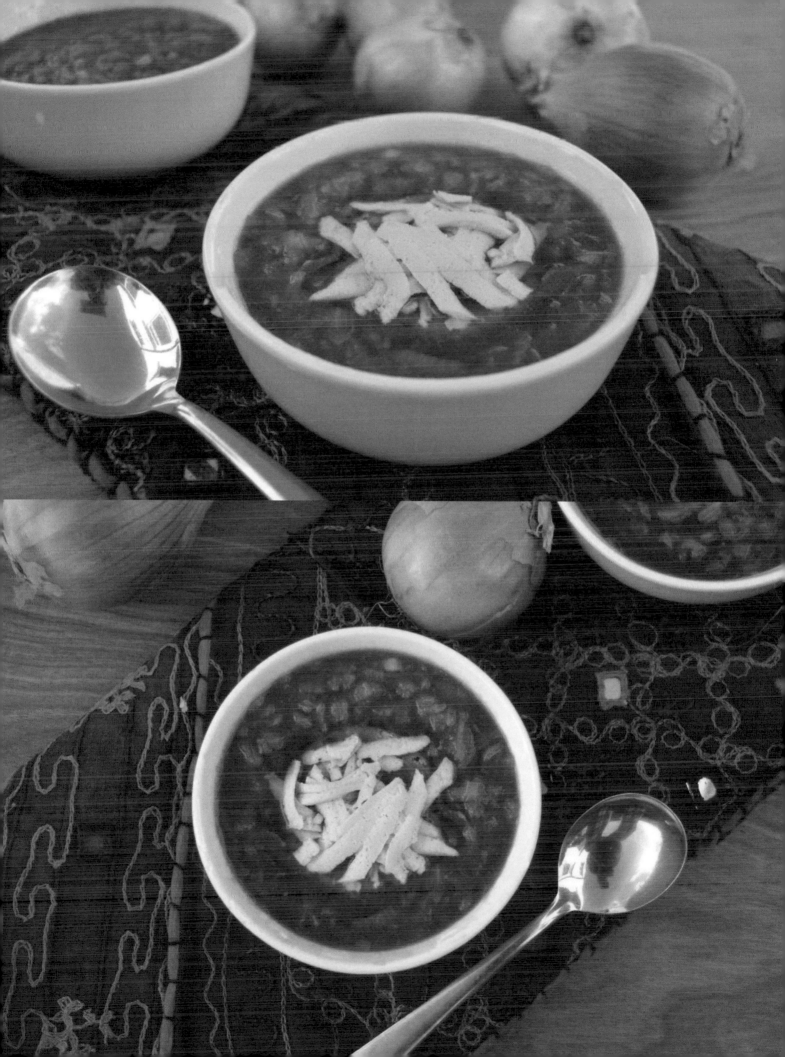

Cauliflower Wings or Burger with Raw Ranch

Makes 4 burgers and 4 servings of wings | 1h 20 mins

This may take over an hour to do, but most of this time is the oven doing all the work. You can either make as small "wing" bites or make as a cauliflower burger. The middle of the cauliflower works best as burgers and you can usually get 4 good slices. I tend to use two cauliflowers and make a batch of both and leave one in the fridge to cook the next day.

Ingredients
- 1 large **Cauliflower**

Chickpea batter (nf)
- 1 tin **Chickpeas**, 15oz / 400ml
- 1 clove **Garlic**
- 1 slice **Red onion**
- 1 tsp **Cumin**
- 1 tsp **Paprika**
- 1 tsp **Turmeric**
- pinch of **Salt** and **Pepper**
- **Water** to blend, about 5 tbsp

Equipment
- Blender
- Oven
- Greaseproof / parchment paper

Raw Ranch Dressing
- 1 cup / 150g **Cashew nuts**
- 1 clove **Garlic**
- 3 tbsp **Apple Cider Vinegar** (page 110)
- handful of **Chives**, chopped
- handful of **Basil leaves**, chopped
- pinch of **Salt** and **Pepper**
- **Water** to blend, about 5 tbsp

Chilli Batter
- 1 tsp dried **Chillies** or cayenne pepper
- 6-8 pitted **Dates**
- 3 tbsp **Apple Cider Vinegar** (page 110)
- 2 tbsp **Olive oil** (optional)
- pinch of **Salt** and **Pepper**

Method
1. Pre heat the oven to 450F / 230C.
2. Put all of the chick pea batter ingredients into a blender and whizz until smooth. You may need to add more water.
3. Chop one medium cauliflower into bite size florets for wings or slices for burgers.
4. Dip all of the cauliflower florets into the chick pea batter and coat. Shake off the excess and place on a non stick sheet and bake for 30 minutes until golden. Toss halfway through.
5. Repeat steps 3 and 4 for the chilli batter to coat the once baked cauliflower again and bake. Again take out of the oven after about 30 minutes once they are golden.
6. To make the ranch dressing blend everything apart from the basil and chives until smooth. Then stir in the chopped herbs and either place in a dipping bowl or on top of the burger.
7. Enjoy immediately or store in the fridge where they will last a few days. The cauliflower wings are best eaten warm.

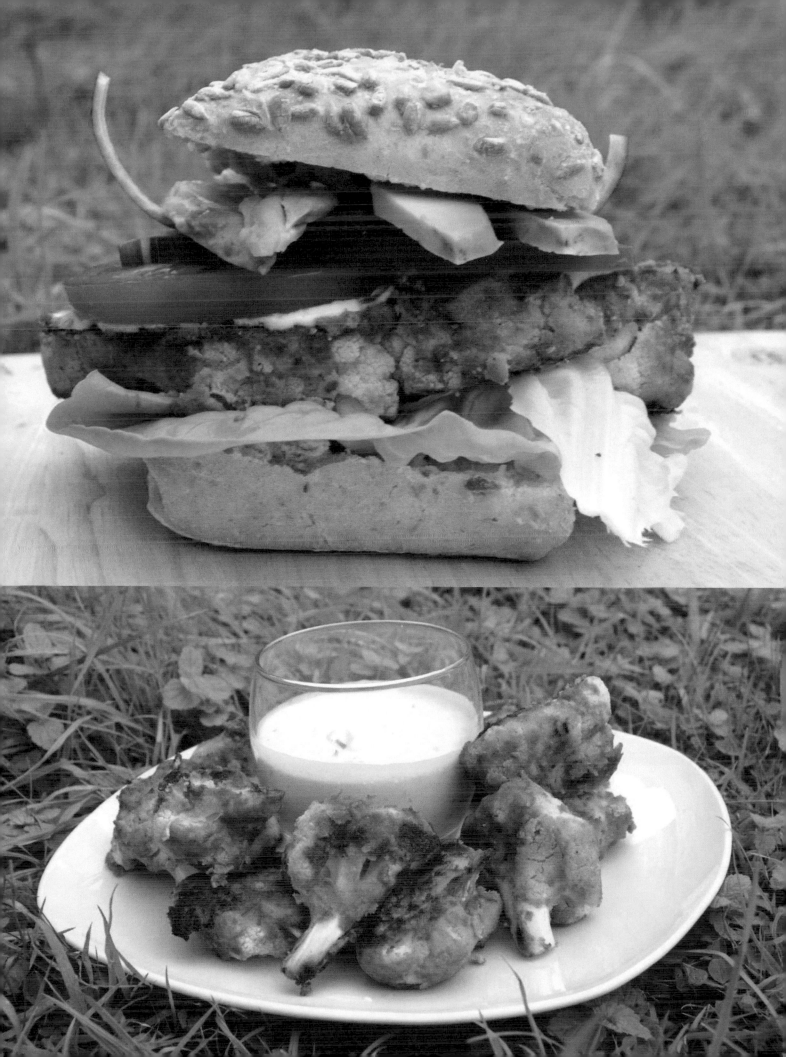

Yeast Extract Cashew Cheese

Makes 10 servings | 10 mins

Easy to make dairy-free cashew based cheese with yeast extract. Most shop bought vegan cheeses are full of unhealthy fats (often unethical palm oil) and low in protein.

This nut cheese contains only the heart-healthy fats from whole cashew nuts and is high in protein. It grates, slices and can be browned under the grill. Yeast extract spreads like marmite and vegemite mean that this vegan cheese contains all B vitamins including the elusive B12.

Ingredients

- 1 cup / 150g **Cashew nuts**
- 1 tbsp **Yeast extract**
- ½ cup / 40g **Nutritional Yeast** (page 108)
- 1 tbsp **Apple Cider Vinegar** (page 110)
- 1 tbsp **Maple syrup**
- 2 cloves **Garlic**
- ¼ tsp **Turmeric**
- ¼ tsp **Cayenne pepper**
- 1½ cups / 350ml **Water**
- 1 tbsp **Agar Agar Powder** (page 94)

Equipment

- Small blender
- Pan
- 5" round tin or bowl
- Greaseproof / parchment paper

Method

1. Place half the water and all the other ingredients (apart from the agar agar) into a small blender and blend until smooth.
2. Bring the other half of the water to a simmer, sprinkle on the agar agar and simmer for 5 minutes while stirring constantly.
3. Take the pan off the heat, stir in the cashew mixture and pour into a dish to set.
4. Chill in the fridge for about 2 hours and it will be set.
5. Enjoy within 5 days and keep in the fridge.

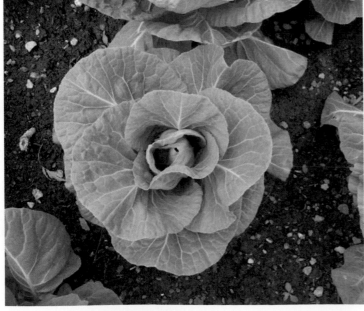

B12

This is one of the few vitamins that is not abundantly available in a vegan diet.

Deficiencies can be serious but luckily it's cheap and safe to ensure you get enough by either having foods fortified with B12 (like yeast extract) or supplementation.

B12 can be found in soil and the micro-organisms it contains. But most commercial produce is pressure washed and this removes any useful source of B12. If you have muddy produce don't worry if a little bit of soil remains as it will possibly do some good.

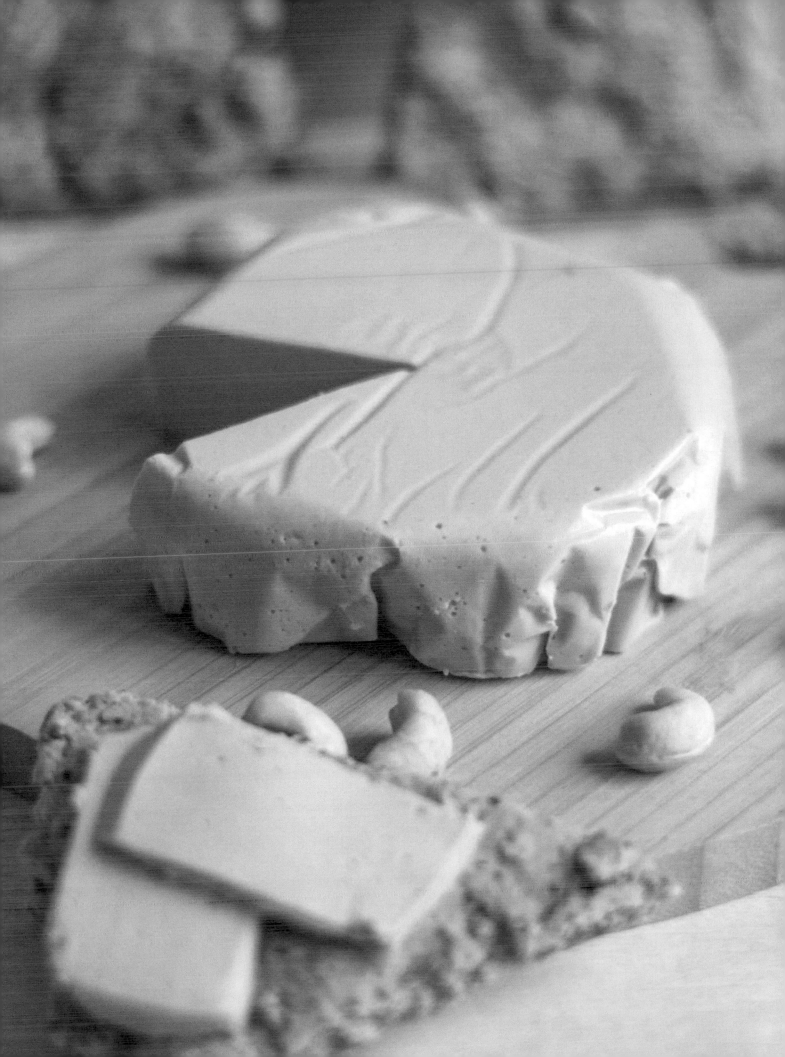

Pistachio Nut Cheese

Makes 10 servings | 10 mins

This quick recipe for dairy-free Pistachio Nut Cheese is easy and foolproof. It slices, grates and will go golden brown when grilled. The only difficult part is not eating the pistachio nuts when making! However it's better to make this cheese than just eat the pistachio nuts as they are sprouted meaning the goodness and nutrients are easily digested.

Ingredients

- 1 cup / 150g **Pistachio nuts**, shelled
- ½ cup / 40g **Nutritional Yeast**
- 1 tbsp **Maple syrup**
- 1 tbsp **Agar Agar Powder** (page 94)
- 2 cloves of **Garlic**
- ½ **Lemon** juiced
- 1 tbsp **Apple Cider Vinegar** (page 110)
- 1½ cups / 350ml **Water**
- 2 pinches of **Salt**

Equipment

- Small blender
- Pan
- 5" round tin or bowl
- Greaseproof / parchment paper - optional but helps make it easy to turn out and gives the wrinkled lines.

Method

1. Soak the pistachio nuts in water with a pinch of salt for an hour or overnight, then drain.
2. Place half the fresh water and everything else apart from the agar agar into a blender.
3. Blend until smooth.
4. In a pan put the remaining half of the water and the agar agar.
5. Simmer for 5 minutes stirring constantly. Make sure no lumps of agar agar form at the bottom.
6. Take off the heat and stir in the pistachio mixture until combined.
7. Pour into a mould and then chill for 2 hours.
8. Enjoy within 3 days and keep chilled.

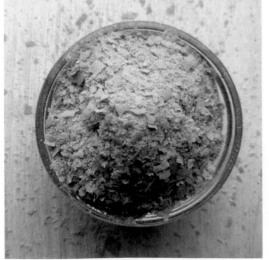

Nutritional Yeast

Nutritional yeast is a savoury vegan food with a cheesy nutty taste. Also known as yeast flakes and nooch. It's very popular in the healthy / raw / vegan world to add the cheesy taste that is difficult to achieve without dairy. It doesn't sound like the most appetising food especially as its best described as looking like fish food. However it is a staple in my kitchen and a delicious versatile ingredient.

As you would expect from the name nutritional yeast it's loaded with nutrients - rich in B vitamins, folic acid, zinc and some brands have added B12.

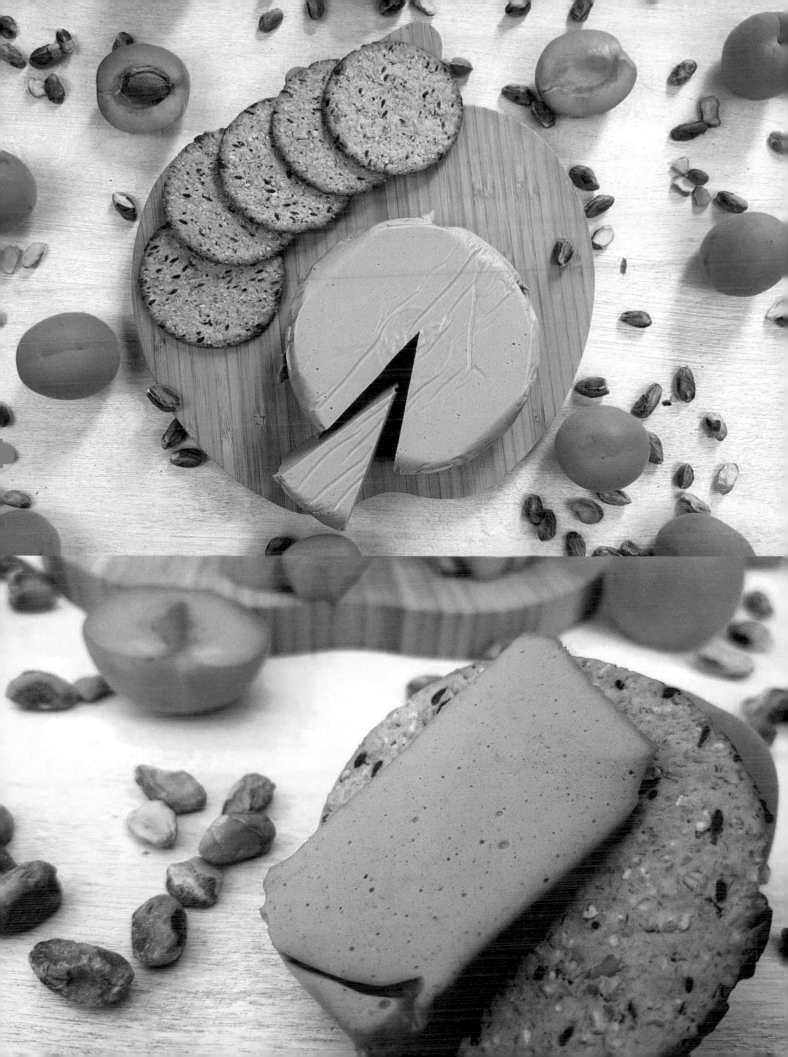

Almond Tomato and Red Pepper Gazpacho

Makes 4 servings | 10 mins

Easy to make raw gazpacho with almonds, red peppers and tomatoes. This recipe is oil free and almonds are added in place of olive oil to give heart-healthy fats and a portion of protein. Perfect light and healthy recipe for a hot summers day to help you cool down.

Ingredients

- 1.5lb / 700g **Tomatoes**
- ½ **Cucumber**
- ¾ cup / 100g **Almonds**
- 2 **Red peppers**
- 3 **Garlic** cloves
- 3 **Spring onions**
- 6 **Sun-dried tomatoes**, optional
- 4 tbsp **Apple Cider Vinegar (page 110)**
- ½ **Red onion**
- 1 tsp **Smoked paprika**
- pinch of **Salt**, optional
- Garnishes – Basil, cucumber, tomato and onion

Equipment

- Blender

Method

1. Soak the almonds in water with a pinch of salt for at least 15 minutes or 8 hours / overnight.
2. Drain the almonds and then add them to a blender along with everything else.
3. You can peel the cucumber if you like, left on does affect the colour but it is more nutritious. I peeled it for the photos for aesthetic reasons only.
4. Blend until the consistency desired is reached. 20 seconds and chunky is how I like it.
5. Chill for an hour then garnish and enjoy within 3 days.

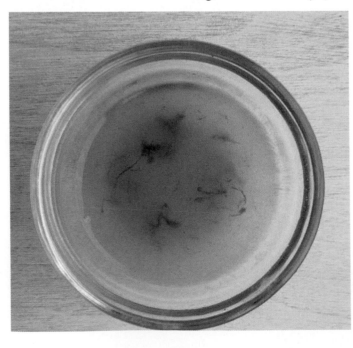

Apple Cider Vinegar

When I refer to apple cider vinegar in this book I always use unpasteurised and unfiltered apple cider with the mother. This may sound like a mouthful but unfiltered and unrefined ACV has more health benefits as it contains a live colony of beneficial bacteria.

You can tell if ACV is unfiltered with the mother as it will have strands of sediment at the bottom.

ACV taken internally can help with digestive problems, boost immunity and balance blood sugar. Externally, when diluted it can help with skin conditions such as sunburn and rashes.

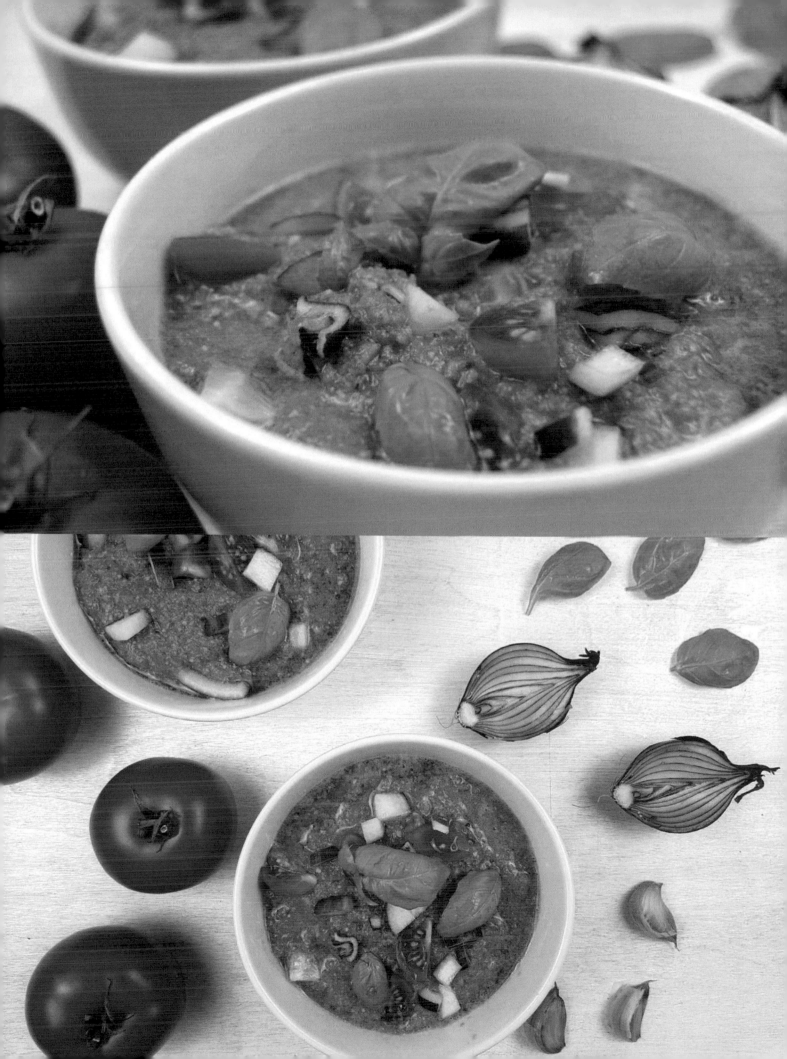

Summer Rolls with Zesty Sauce

Makes 12 half rolls | 30 mins

These summer rolls are fun to make and look very tempting. They are filled with a rainbow of fresh raw fruit and vegetables. You can use any fruit or veg that you have – the only ingredient I always add is avocado.

Some people avoid peanuts and the sauce can be made with any other nut or seed butter. I've made it with cashew butter, almond butter and raw sunflower seed and all have turned out great.

Ingredients (nf)

- 6 sheets **Vietnamese rice paper**
- **Lettuce**
- **Avocado**
- **Mango**
- **Carrot**
- **Cucumber**
- **Red pepper**
- **Red cabbage**
- **Coriander / Cilantro**
- **Spring onion**
- **Raspberries**

Zesty Nut/Seed Lemon Sauce

- 2 tbsp **Peanut or Almond butter,** – or any other nut / seed butter
- 1 tsp **Soy sauce / Tamari**
- 1 **Lemon**, juiced
- 1 clove **Garlic**, finely chopped
- 1 tsp **Cayenne pepper**
- 2 tbsp **Water**

Method

1. Chop all fruit and vegetables into thin strips, apart from small fruit like berries.
2. Dip a sheet of rice paper in warm water for a few seconds.
3. Remove from the water when it begins to soften but still has some shape.
4. Place flat on a board and then add thin slices of fruit and vegetables on 1/3 of the paper at an edge.
5. Roll the rice paper up by folding over the filling, tucking in the sides then rolling to the edge. See the video at nestandglow.com for a demo.
6. Mix all of the satay ingredients together until they are combined. You may want to add more / less cayenne pepper depending on how spicy you like it.
7. Slice all of the rolls in the middle and enjoy by dipping in the sauce.
8. They will last a few days in the fridge.

Rainbow Diet

Foods of different colours contains different vitamins and minerals. An easy way to make sure you get a good range of vitamins, minerals and other nutrients is to eat a rainbow of different coloured foods. However you don't have to have all of the rainbow in every meal.

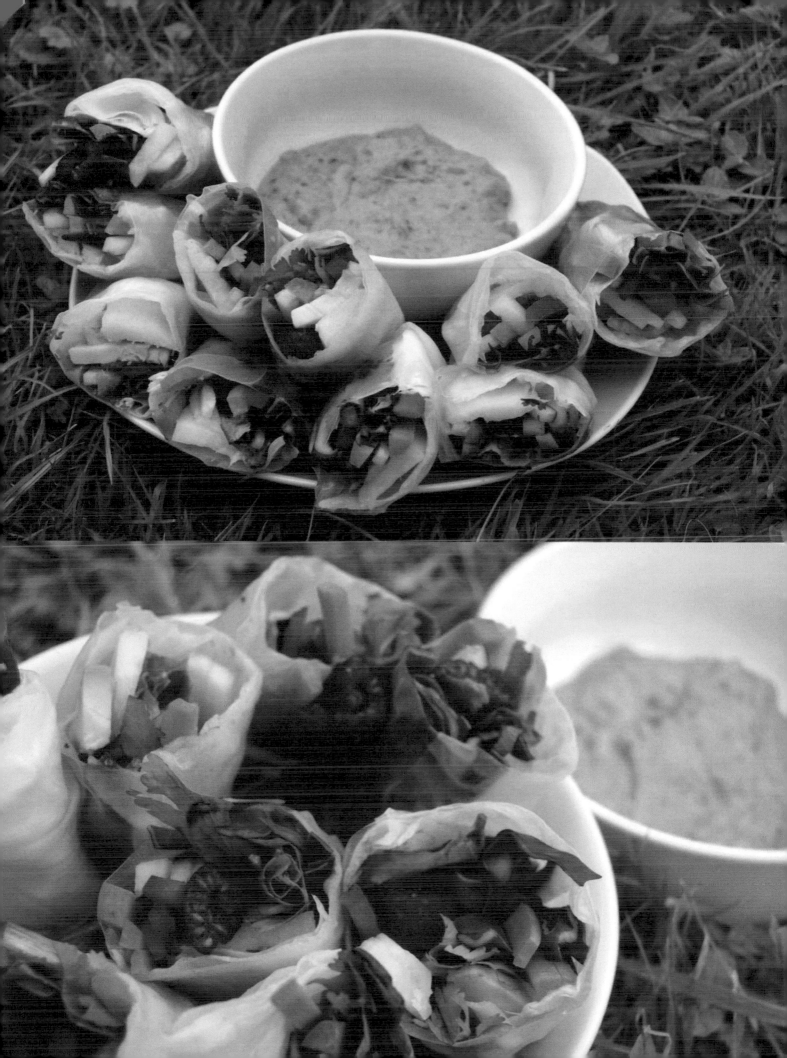

Roasted Butternut Squash Almond Soup

Serves 4 | 1h (p)

Easy to make creamy roasted butternut squash and almond soup. Perfect for a cold winter's day to warm you up. It's very mildly spiced so if you like your curry I would recommend doubling all the spices.

This may sound like a lot of work and difficult, but like all of my recipes it's pretty easy. Simply cut the butternut in half and then roast for an hour. Then when it's done scoop out the flesh and simmer. It's actually less work than peeling the squash and roasted butternut tastes great.

Ingredients

- 1 **Butternut squash**
- 2 large **Onions**
- 2 cloves **Garlic**
- ½ tsp **Cayenne pepper**
- ½ tsp **Turmeric**
- ½ tsp **Cumin**
- 4 cups / 1L **Vegetable stock**
- 2 tbsp **Almond butter**, or any other nut / seed butter
- 1 tbsp **Pumpkin seeds**

Equipment

- Stick hand blender
- Saucepan

Method

1. Cut the butternut in half, no need to remove the stem, scoop out the seeds and dry bake (no oil needed) for 1 hour at 450F / 230C. Check half way through that it isn't burning.
2. Scoop out all of the butternut flesh. Don't bin the skins they have lots of nutrients and can be placed back in the oven for a chefs treat.
3. Peel and dice the onions and garlic. Then cook on a high heat with a dash of water for 5 minutes until translucent.
4. Add everything else and simmer for 5 minutes then take off the heat, blend and serve.
5. Sprinkle with pumpkin and cumin seeds for extra flavour and crunch. Enjoy immediately.

Butternut and Sweet Potato Skins

I usually bake my butternut and sweet potato whole as it saves any pealing but also because then you get the chefs treat of the skins. After baking the flesh comes away easily enough and the skins can be enjoyed as they are or placed back in the oven to crisp up a bit more. These taste great drizzled in vinegar and a sprinkle of salt. The seeds of a butternut are also delicious after being roasted - eat the whole thing including the outer husk.

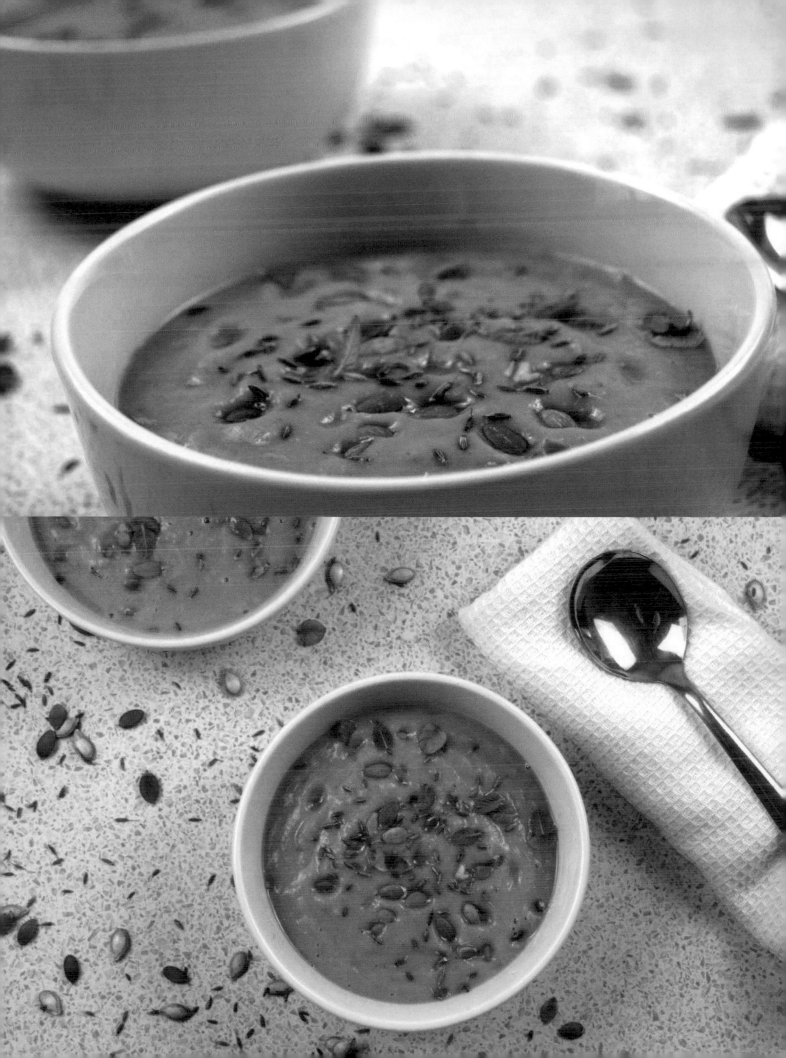

Sushi Spring Buns with Spicy Almond Dip

Makes 12 buns | 45 mins

These easy to make sushi spring roll buns are a mixture of summer rolls and sushi with seasoned brown rice and seaweed. They look very tempting with a fan of avocado, orange carrots, red cabbage with a spicy and zesty raw almond dip. Perfect as a side dish or a main meal as they are loaded with vegetables, complex carbohydrates and heart healthy fats from the almonds and avocado.

Ingredients

- 12 sheets of **Rice paper**
- 2 **Avocados**, sliced finely lengthways
- 2 **Carrots**, julienned
- 2-4 tbsp **Seaweed** – any you like such as dulse, sea lettuce or nori
- ¼ **Red cabbage**, finely sliced
- **Sesame seeds**, to sprinkle on top

Seasoned Sushi Brown Rice

- 1 cup / 190g **Brown rice**, uncooked
- 2 tbsp rice or **Apple Cider Vinegar (page 110)**
- 2 tbsp **Maple** or rice Syrup
- 2 tbsp **Sesame seeds**

Spicy and Zesty Almond Dip

- 1 cup / 140g **Almonds**, soaked
- 1-2 cloves of **Garlic**, peeled
- 1 tsp, **Cayenne pepper**
- 2 **Lemons**, juice of
- A pinch of **Salt**
- **Water**, just enough for blending

Equipment

- Blender
- Bowl of warm water

Method

1. Soak the almonds in water for at least 15 minutes, overnight is best.
2. Cook the brown rice, then set aside for 10 minutes to cool.
3. Mix all of the seasoned rice ingredients together, use a plastic or metal spoon to prevent the rice breaking up.
4. Slice and prep all the filling ingredients.
5. Soak a sheet of rice paper in warm water for a few seconds, then fan out 5 or so slices of avocado in the middle then top with vegetables, seaweed and rice.
6. Fold the rice paper to the top and going around in a circle fold about every 1/8th. Pinch the rice paper together at the top and then lay down fold side down. There is a video demonstration of this at nestandglow.com.
7. Drain the almonds then place with all the other dip ingredients and blend until smooth. Add as little water as possible.
8. Ready to eat straight away but will last a few days in the fridge.

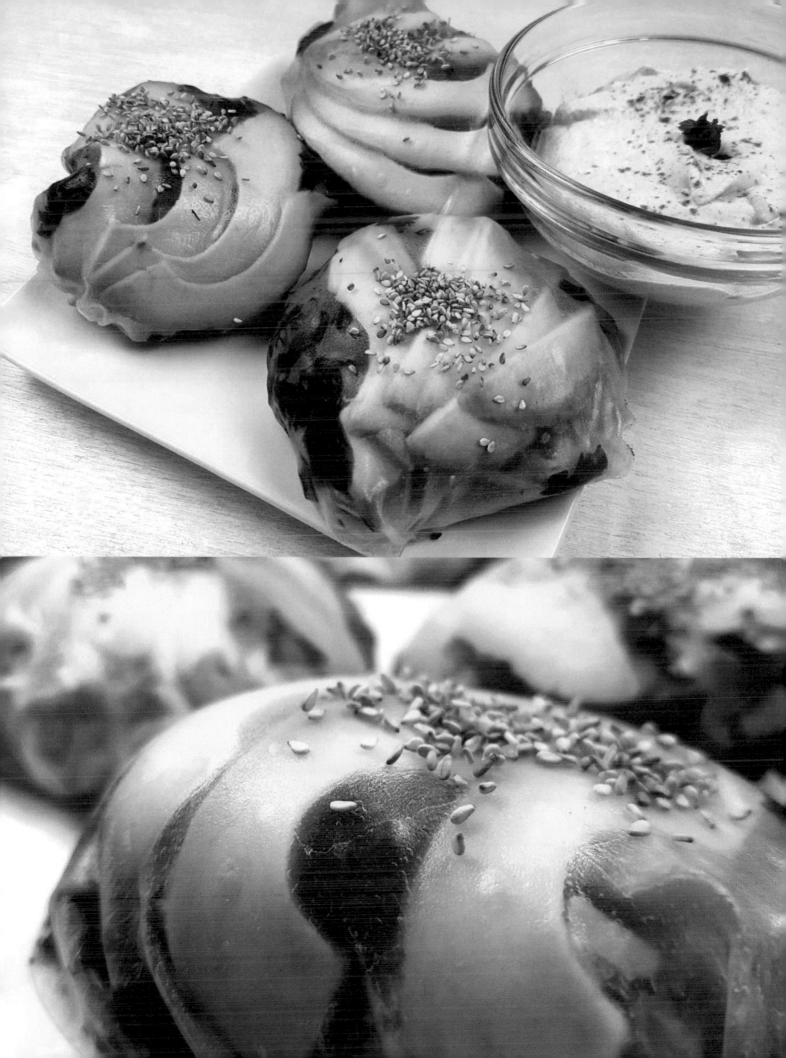

Cheesy Kale Crisps

Makes 8 servings | 40 mins baked | 10.5h raw

Kale crisps are a ridiculously healthy and delicious alternative to deep fried potato crisps. You can make these kale crisps raw using a Dehydrator (page 36) or baked with a oven. Both of these varieties are high in protein and a source of iron, calcium and vitamins A, C and K.

Ingredients for Both

- 1 cup / 140g **Sunflower seeds**
- 14oz / 400g **Kale**, still on stems
- 4 tbsp **Nutritional Yeast** (page 108)
- 2 cloves of **Garlic**
- 2 tbsp **Apple Cider Vinegar** (page 110)
- pinch of **Salt** and **Pepper**
- ½ cup / 120ml **Water**
- **Water** and pinch of **Salt** for soaking

Smoked Sun Cheese Kale Crisps

- 1 tbsp **Smoked paprika**
- ¼ tsp **Turmeric**
- ¼ tsp **Cayenne pepper**
- 4 **Dates**, pitted

Cheese and Onion Kale Crisps

- 1 small **Onion**
- 2 tbsp **Virgin olive oil**, optional

Equipment

- Blender, Oven/Dehydrator, greaseproof paper

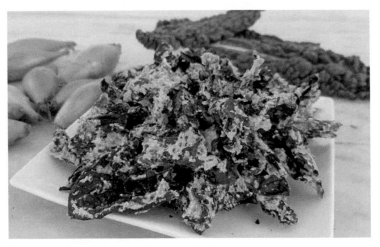

Method

1. Soak the sunflower seeds in water with a pinch of salt. Overnight is best.
2. Rip the kale off the stems. Remove up to where the stem snaps.
3. Place the kale in a bowl and sprinkle over a pinch of salt and the apple cider vinegar.
4. Scrunch the kale up using your hands until it's halved in volume.
5. Drain the sunflower seeds and place with all the other ingredients into a blender then blend until smooth. Add the base ingredients and the additional ingredients for each flavour.
6. Pour the sunflower sauce onto the kale and massage to coat all the leaves.
7. Baked or Raw:
   - **Bake**; spread out thinly onto a lined tray and bake at 300F / 150C for about 25-30 minutes. Toss every 5-10 minutes and take out of the oven as soon as they are dry. Watch like a hawk as they burn easily.
   - **Raw**; spread out thinly on to a non-stick sheet. Dry at 110C / 43C for 10-12 hours tossing half way.
8. Enjoy the kale crisps straight after cooking / drying.
9. Once cooled they can be stored in an airtight container for a few weeks, but it's best to have them the same day as they loose their crispiness.

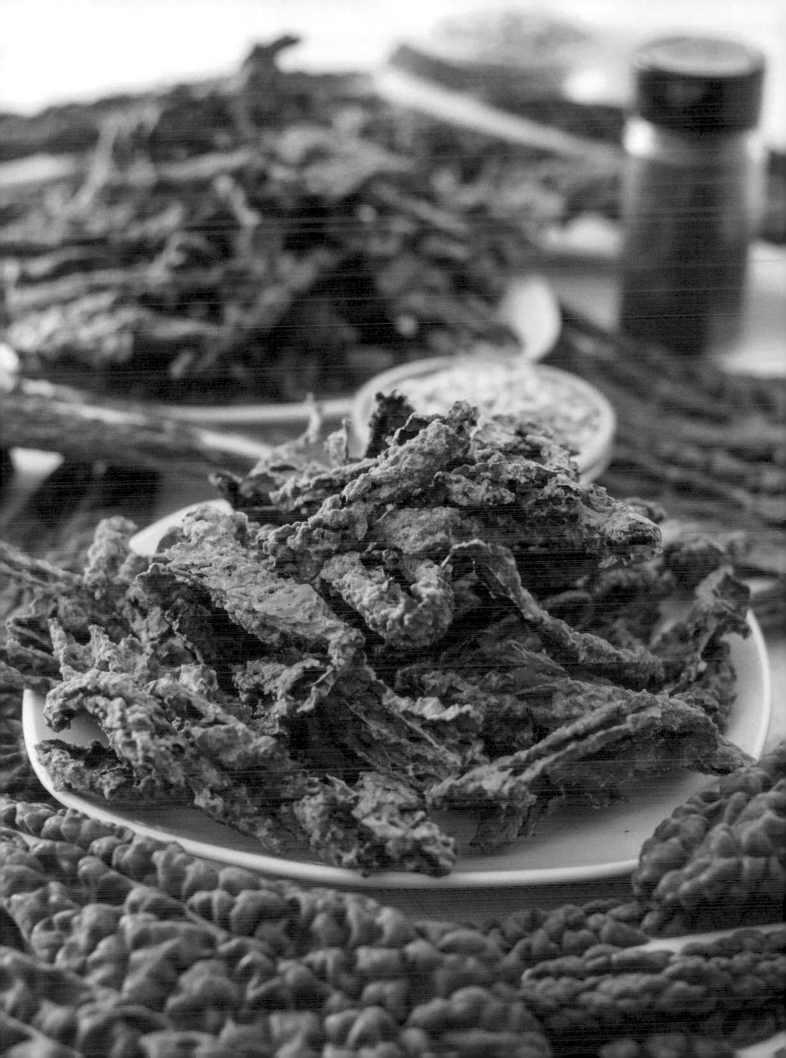

Tomato and Basil Lentil Chips

Makes 6 servings | 1h 20 mins **nf**

These healthy baked chips are high protein and free of oil, nuts, seeds and grains.

The lentil chips have a sweet tangy tomato base with a hint of aromatic basil. They are very inexpensive to make and are crispy, filling, high in fibre and vitamins. What isn't there to love about these chips?

Ingredients

- 1 cup / 140g **Red split lentils**
- 4 tbsp **Tomato puree**
- 1 slice **Onion**
- 2 cloves **Garlic**
- 1 tsp **Smoked paprika**
- ½ tsp **Turmeric**
- ½ tsp **Cayenne pepper**
- 2 tbsp **Apple Cider Vinegar** (page 110)
- 1 tbsp **Maple syrup**
- pinch of **Salt** and **Pepper**
- ¾ cup / 180ml **Water**
- 1 tbsp dried **Basil**

Equipment

- Blender
- Oven
- Greaseproof / parchment paper

Greaseproof / Parchment paper

These two types of paper are the same. I use this paper a lot for baked recipes in this book as they make it easy to take something gluten-free out of a pan easily without needing to oil the pan.

Do not use wax paper in these baking recipes as it's not heat resistant.

Method

1. Soak the lentils in salted water for at least an hour, overnight is best.
2. Drain and rinse the lentils then add to a blender with everything else apart from the basil.
3. Blend until smooth.
4. Pour on to a greaseproof paper lined baking dish and spread to the sides and sprinkle on the dried basil.
5. If you have a dish that fills a normal oven then this will make one batch, for a half size mini oven like I use it makes two batches.
6. Bake at 375F / 190C for 30 minutes.
7. Remove from the oven and let stand for 10 minutes.
8. Peel off the greaseproof paper and cut into long strips, then into triangles. One batch makes about 50 chips.
9. Place directly on an oven wire rack then bake for another 20-30 minutes at 375F / 190C.
10. Remove from the oven when the edges are golden.
11. Enjoy as soon as they are out of the oven, or keep chilled in an airtight container for up to 3 days.

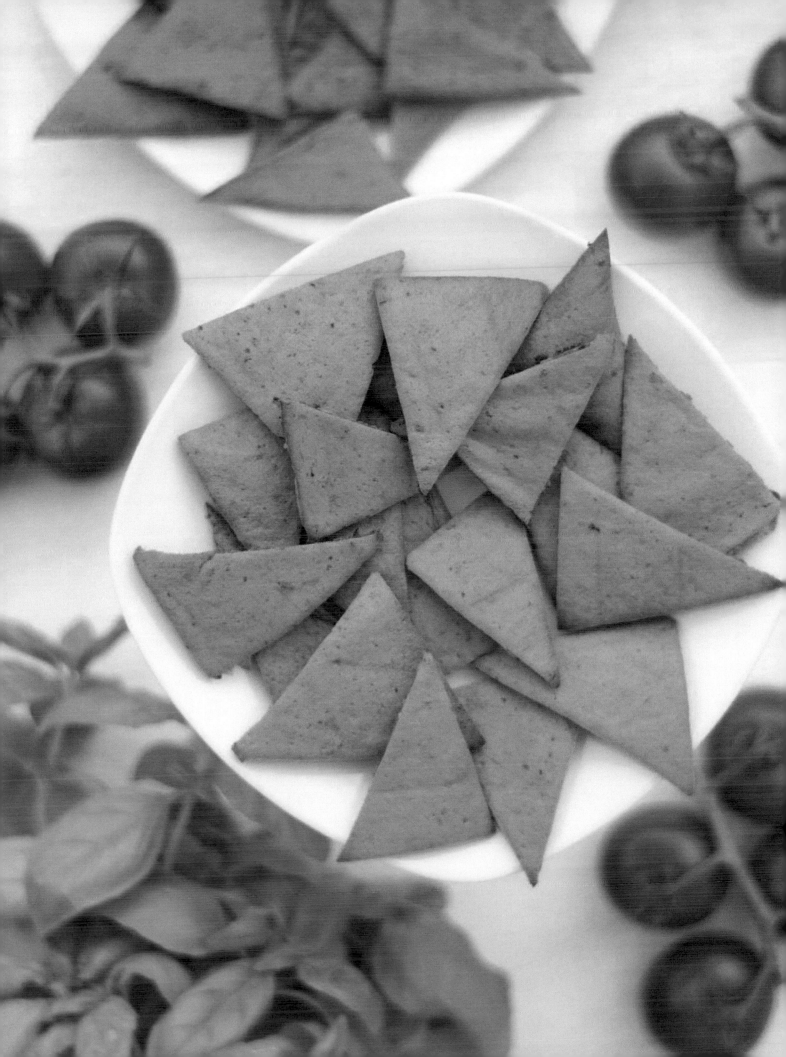

Kale Crunch Salad

Makes 4 servings | 15 mins

Try this easy recipe to get all the goodness of kale in a delicious tasty side dish, infinitely tastier than boiled spinach. The kale is slightly steamed in order to break down the cell walls and make it easy to absorb. It has a salty sweet dressing from maple syrup and soy sauce but you can replace either of these with something sweet / salty. Replace the soy with something salty to make paleo.

Ingredients

- 2-3 heads of **Kale**
- 1 tbsp **Maple syrup**
- 1 tbs **Soy sauce / Miso / Tamari**
- 2 tbsp **Sesame seeds**
- 5 **Radishes**
- 1 small **Carrot**, cut into ribbons
- a few slices of **Red cabbage**

Equipment

- Steamer and Bowl

Method

1. Rip the kale off its stalks and slice into bite size strips.
2. Steam the kale for 3-4 minutes until tender.
3. Put the kale in a bowl and sprinkle on the soy sauce and maple syrup.
4. Finely slice the red cabbage and radish. Use a vegetable peeler to make carrot ribbons.
5. Sprinkle on the cabbage, carrot, radish, and sesame seeds and serve immediately.

Tamari

This is a Japanese soy sauce that is typically wheat-free unlike many soy sauces. Do however still check the label to ensure that it's wheat and gluten-free.

It has a richer and deeper flavour so you use less compared to normal soy sauce. Tamari is a by product of miso production.

Traditional soy sauce is Chinese and is brewed rather than fermented.

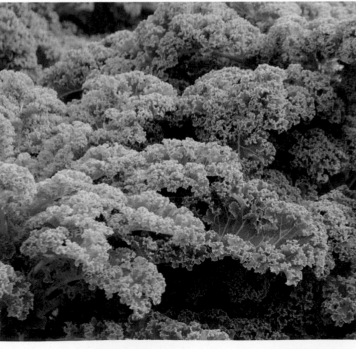

Leafy Greens

Dark green leafy vegetables are very nutrient dense and full of vitamins and minerals. I have a vegan vitamins and minerals chart in my kitchen to remind me to eat a wide variety of produce and leafy greens are the one food type that shows up in most of the vitamins and minerals columns.

Leafy Green Vegetables:

Kale, Chard, Broccoli, Spinach, Rocket, Mustard Greens, Bok Choy, Watercress, Spring/Collard Greens, Turnip Greens, Dandelion Leaves, Mint, Basil, Coriander & Parsley.

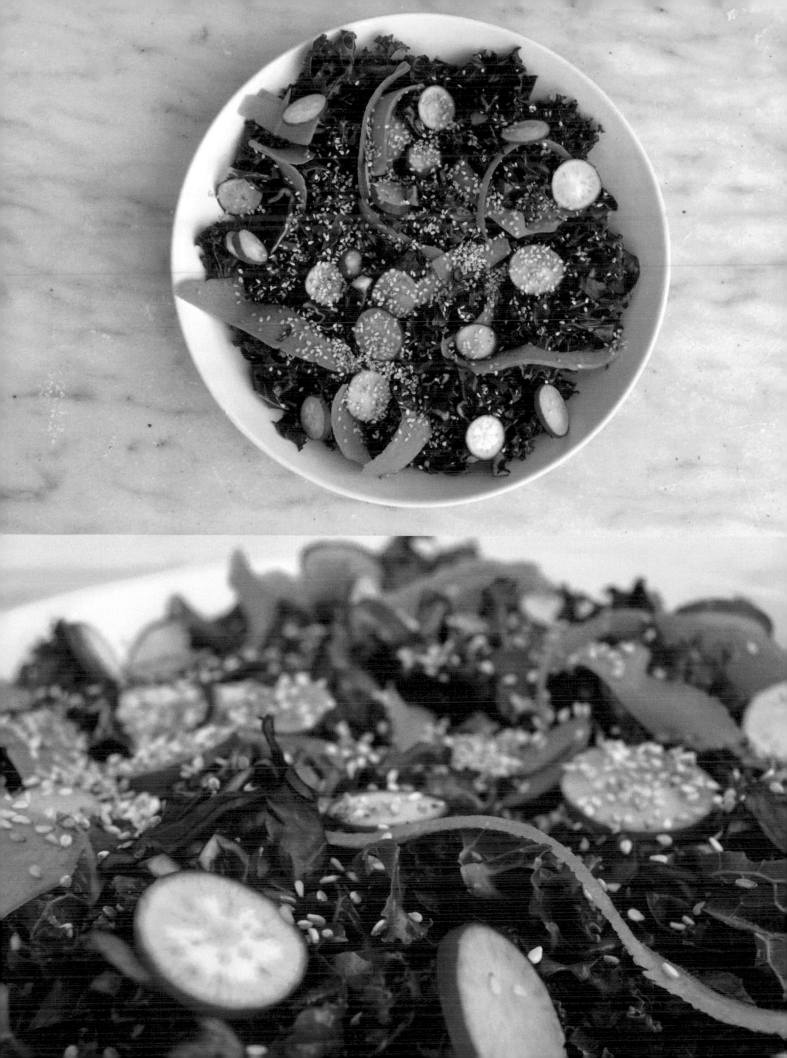

Almond Milk and Almond Cheese

Makes 2 pints & 4 cheese balls | 10 mins **raw** **p**

Almond milk and cheese is easy to make and homemade tastes much better than shop bought. This version is nutritionally superior with a high almond content and a healthy dose of protein. The almonds are sprouted to aid absorption. Most commercial almond milks contain very little almond (often less than 1%) and a host of other additives and stabilisers.

Ingredients
- 1½ cups / 200g **Almonds**

Almond milk
- 4 cups / 1L **Water**
- ½ tsp **Salt**
- 1 tsp **Vanilla**
- 2 tbs **Sweetener**, Maple syrup or similar

Equipment
- Blender
- Sieve / cheesecloth / nut milk bag

Almond Cheese
- 3 tbsp **Nutritional Yeast** (page 108)
- 1½ tbsp **Coconut oil / butter,** optional
- 1 **Lemon**, juiced
- ½ tsp **Garlic powder**
- ¼ tsp **Salt**
- ¼ tsp **Turmeric**
- ¼ tsp **Cayenne pepper**

Method

1. Soak the almonds in salted water for 8 hours or overnight to sprout them. If you are short of time then a 1-hour soak is acceptable but less than ideal for maximum nutritional benefit.
2. Drain and rinse the almonds then place in a blender with fresh water.
3. Blend for a few minutes.
4. Pour into a cheesecloth, nut bag or sieve and squeeze out the milk.
5. Stir in the vanilla and sweetener to the milk, if desired.
6. Empty the pulp into a bowl with all the other cheese ingredients.
7. Mix together then roll into portion sized balls and chill.
8. Enjoy the cheese and milk within 3 days and store in the fridge.

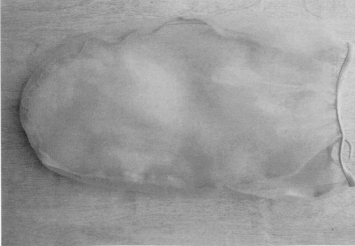

Nut Milk Bags

These are just small bags that are usually made out of nylon. They make separating a liquid from a pulp easy work and are quick to clean under running water. One well cared bag will last for years.

You can make your own if you're handy or use a cheesecloth instead.

See "Seed Milks" on page 172 and "Blender Juicing" on page 28.

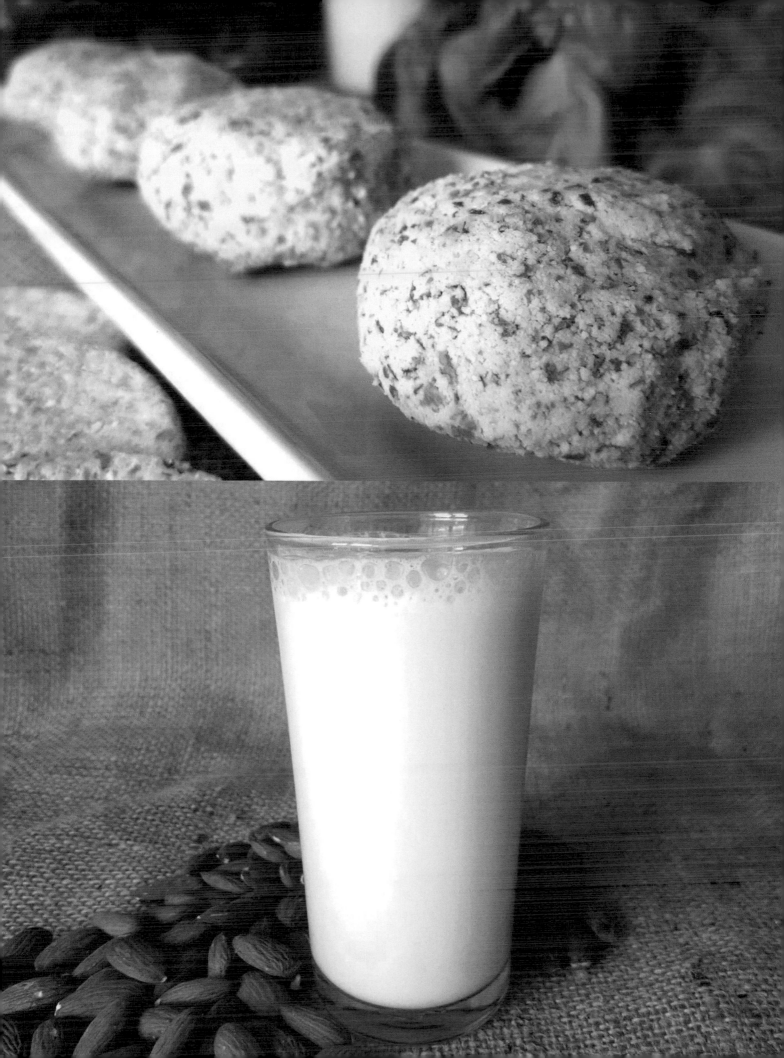

Fruity & Nutty Cauliflower Crunch

Makes 4 servings | 20 mins **raw** **p**

Fruity and nutty cauliflower 'couscous' crunch with a curry maple dressing. This salad looks very appetising and tastes great with red pomegranate, orange apricots and green pistachios. Perfect for summer days and great to bring along to picnics or barbecues.

Ingredients

- 1 **Cauliflower**, stem removed and broken into florets
- 1 tbsp **Curry powder**
- 1 tbsp **Maple syrup** / other sweetener,
- 3 tbsp **Apple Cider Vinegar** (page 110)
- 3 medium **Spring onions**
- 4 **Apricots**, diced
- 1 tbsp **Tamari / soy sauce /** pinch **Salt** (P)

- 1 **Pomegranate**, seeds of
- 100g / ¾ cup **Pistachios**, raw and unshelled
- 60g / ⅓ cup **Hazelnuts**
- 1 bunch **Mint**, fresh
- 1 bunch of **Coriander**, fresh

Equipment

- Food processor

Method

1. Pulse blend the cauliflower in a food processor until it's broken up into couscous sized pieces. It doesn't matter if there are a few large pieces but you want to avoid over blending and making it mushy.
2. Mix together the curry powder, maple syrup and apple cider vinegar together. Then mix this with the cauliflower couscous.
3. Roughly chop the spring onions, nuts and herbs and then mix everything together and serve.
4. Ready to eat straight away or it will last a few days when stored in the fridge.

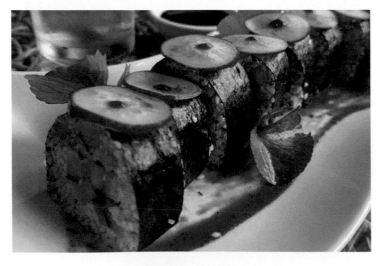

Cauliflower and Parsnip Raw Rice

You can make a raw alternative to rice using cauliflower or parsnip.

Simply place chunks of either in a food processor and pulse blend until broken up into small pieces. Then mix in a pinch of salt, ground sesame seeds, a dash of Apple Cider Vinegar (page 110) and optionally a drizzle of olive oil. Perfect on the side of a curry or to make raw sushi.

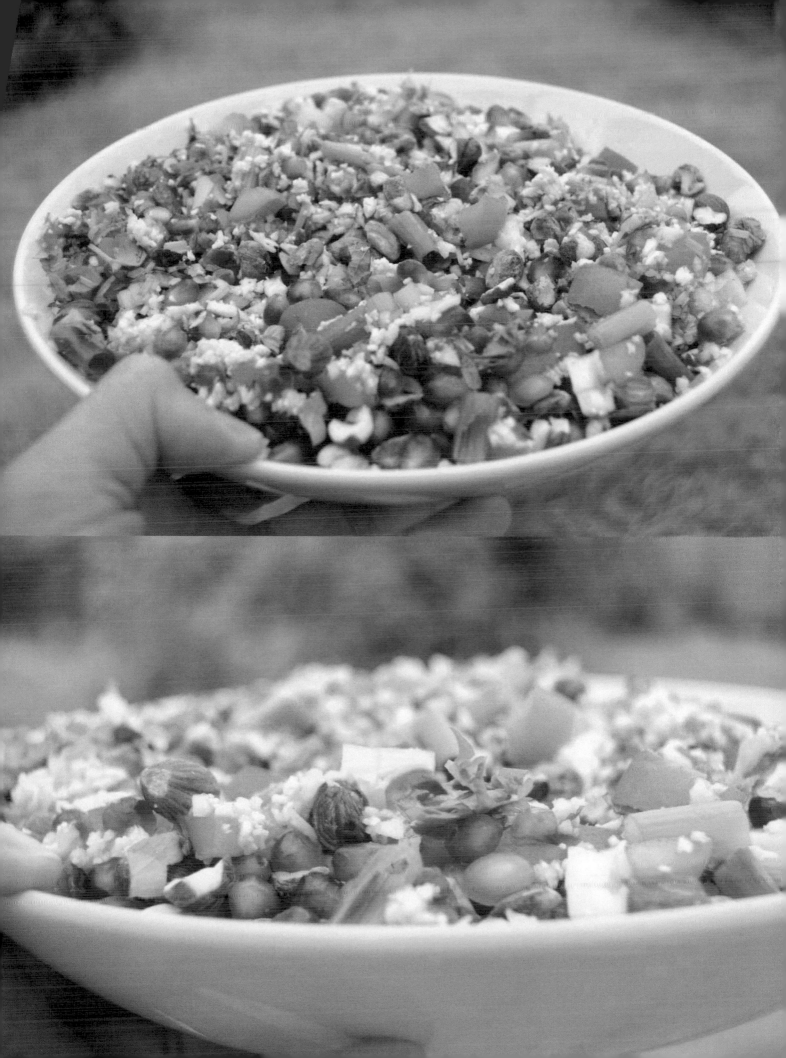

Hummus Trio – Red Pepper, Mint Pea and Beetroot Cumin

Makes 15 servings | 15 mins

Easy recipes for delicious hummus that is flavoured with caramelised roasted red peppers, beetroot cumin and minted peas. These recipes are simple but beautiful with natural bright colours.

I use ground sesame seeds instead of tahini in my hummus, this makes it cheaper and healthier as the seeds have not been roasted at high temperature. Use a coffee grinder to grind up the sesame seeds or a small blender jug.

Base Hummus

- 1 can **Chickpeas**
- 2 tbsp ground **Sesame seeds / Tahini**
- 2 cloves **Garlic**
- 1 **Lemon**, juiced
- ¼ tsp **Turmeric**
- ¼ tsp **Cayenne pepper**
- **Salt** and **Pepper**, to taste
- ½ cup / 120ml **Water**

Mint and Pea Hummus

- 1 cup **Peas**
- 1 handful of **Mint leaves**

Beetroot Cumin Hummus

- 1 tsp **Cumin seeds**
- 4 cooked **Beetroot**

Caramelised Red Onion and Pepper

- 2 **Red peppers**
- 1 **Red onion**
- 1 tbsp **Raisins** / currants

Equipment

- Blender
- Oven
- Greaseproof / parchment paper

Method

1. Put everything from the base recipe into a food processor then either blend to enjoy a normal hummus or add the special ingredients to make a flavoured hummus.

- **Mint and pea hummus:**
  - Either use frozen thawed peas or cook fresh peas and then blend with the mint and base hummus until smooth.
- **Roast red pepper hummus:**
  - Halve two red peppers and remove the stem and seeds.
  - Halve and skin one red onion.
  - Bake on a non-stick sheet for an hour at 250 F / 120C until caramelised and cooked. A few charred bits are fine.
  - Blend the cooked pepper, raisins and onion with the base hummus.
- **Beetroot hummus:**
  - Blend the cooked beetroot and cumin seeds with the base ingredients.

The hummus made will keep for a few days in the fridge.

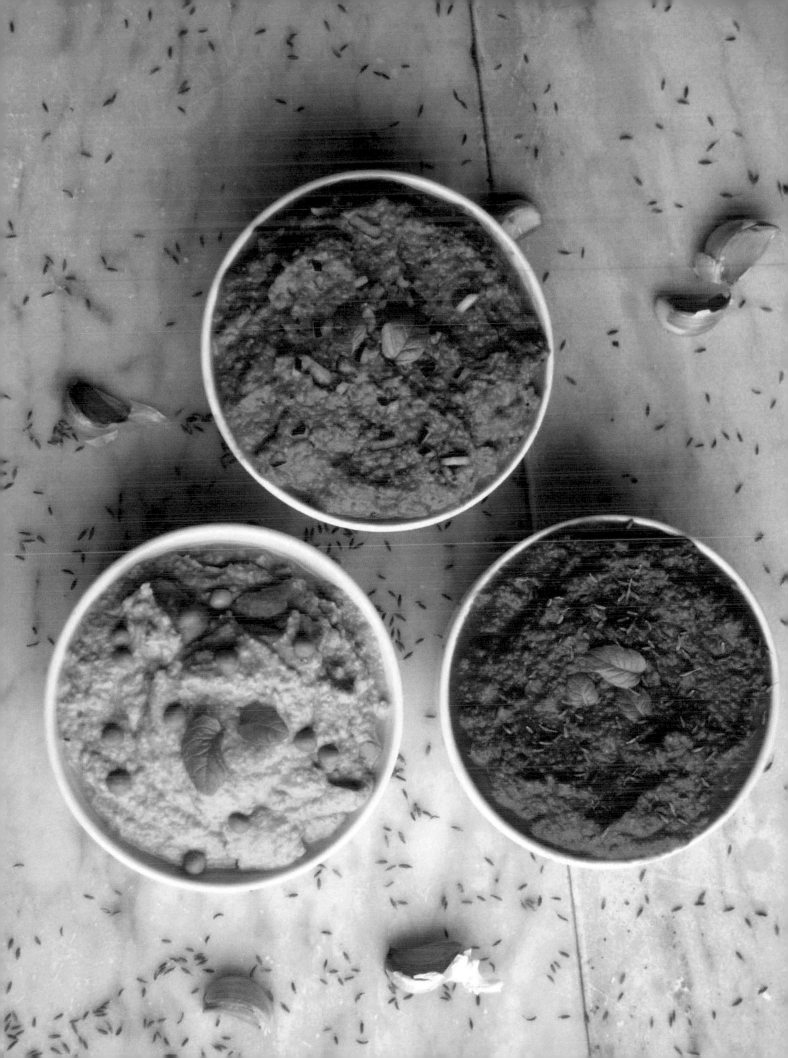

Sweet Potato Quinoa Cinnamon Bites

Makes 15 servings | 15 mins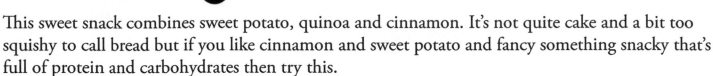

This sweet snack combines sweet potato, quinoa and cinnamon. It's not quite cake and a bit too squishy to call bread but if you like cinnamon and sweet potato and fancy something snacky that's full of protein and carbohydrates then try this.

Perfect on its own or topped with a healthy sweet or savoury spread.

Ingredients

- 2 small **Sweet Potatoes**, about 10oz / 300g
- 1 cup / 175g **Quinoa**
- ½ cup / 120ml **Water**
- 1 tsp **Cinnamon**
- ¼ tsp **Turmeric**
- ¼ tsp **Cayenne pepper**
- pinch of **Salt and pepper**
- ½ tsp **Baking powder**
- **Water** for soaking

Equipment

- Blender
- Oven
- Baking pan 10"
- Greaseproof / parchment paper

Method

1. Soak the quinoa in water for at least 15 minutes, overnight is best.
2. Drain the quinoa and put in a blender with everything apart from the sweet potatoes.
3. Blend until all broken up.
4. Grate the sweet potatoes.
5. Mix everything together and press tightly into a lined pan about 10" square.
6. Bake for about an hour at 350F / 180C until the sweet potato is cooked.
7. Take out of the oven and leave to cool and firm up.
8. Slice into 16 small squares.
9. Eat within 3 days and store in the fridge.

Notes

Leave the skins on the sweet potatoes for maximum nutrition.

This will still be soft when it's taken out of the oven as it's gluten free and will firm up once cooled.

My favourite way to eat these is with the "Avocado Chocolate Icing" on page 4.

To make these more of a savoury snack omit the cinnamon.

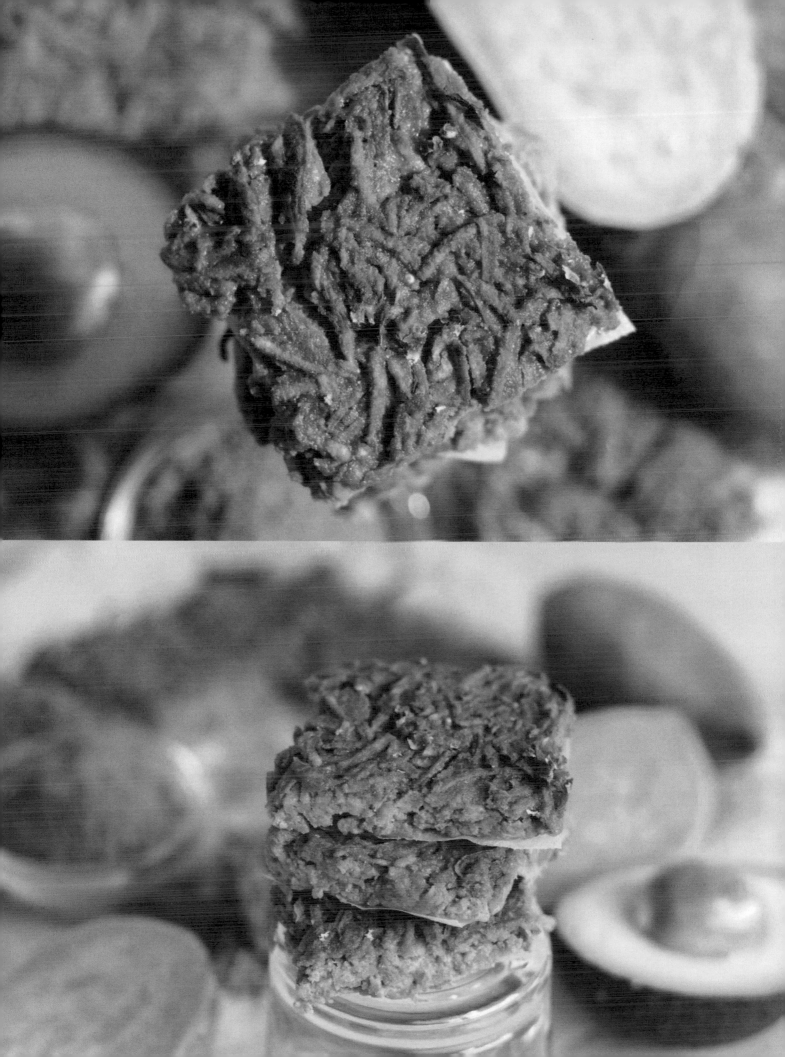

Winter Rolls & Raw Sweet Chilli Dip

Makes 12 half rolls | 15 mins

Think of summer rolls but with autumnal produce and a spicy dip. A rainbow of winter fruit and vegetables with a fresh zesty sauce and plenty of fire from chilli, ginger and garlic.

These are easy to make and are a great starter or party food. You can use any vegetables that you have about, just try to get a rainbow of colours. In the winter I like to have something like this in place of a salad as when its cold eating raw veggies can be unappealing.

Ingredients
- 6 sheets **Rice paper wrappers**

Filling examples
- **Kale**, stem removed
- **Red cabbage**, finely sliced
- **Carrot**, thin strips
- **Bean sprouts**
- **Radish**, thin slices
- **Chives**
- **Mint leaves**
- **Pomegranate seeds**

Raw Sweet Chilli Sauce
- 4-6 pitted **Dates**
- 1 clove **Garlic**
- half a medium **Chilli pepper**, remove the seeds to make it mild
- half an inch of **Ginger**, diced
- juice of 1 **Lime**
- 1 tbsp **Soy sauce / Tamari**
- 2 tbsp **Apple Cider Vinegar** (page 110)
- 1 tbsp **Sesame oil** (optional)

Equipment
- Blender

Method
1. Prepare all the fillings so that they are in small slices / strips that are suitable for the rolls.
2. Dip a sheet of rice paper in warm water for a few seconds.
3. Place the rice paper down on a flat surface and then fill 1/3 of one side with your fruit and veggies. Don't put too much in else it will spill out when rolling.
4. Then roll up like a burrito – roll over the filling, wrap in the sides and continue to roll to the end. See the video recipe at nestandglow.com for a demo.
5. Slice the roll in half at a 45 degree angle and place on serving dish.
6. Put all of the sweet chilli sauce ingredients into a blender and then blend until smooth.
7. Enjoy immediately or store in the fridge where they will last for a day or so.

Raw Coconut Wraps (raw)

I'm using standard rice paper wrappers for the rolls here. You can however use coconut wrappers if you prefer. These can be made by blending young coconut meat with water to make a smooth paste that is dehydrated overnight until firm.

Some health food shops sell these coconut wraps pre-done. There are also varieties with a pinch of turmeric.

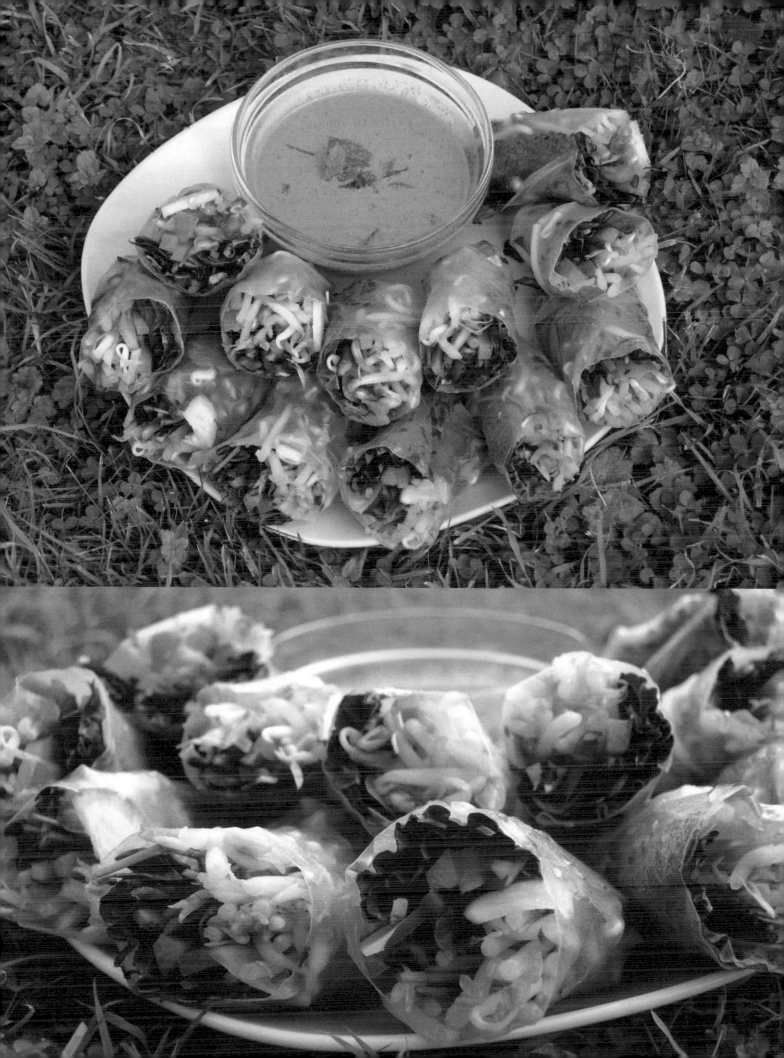

Five Seed Oatcakes

Makes 8 oatcake triangles | 1h 20 mins

These oatcakes are made with a mixture of five different seeds that add taste, crunch and nutrition. Oatcakes are so easy to make that you will wonder why you ever used to buy them! These oatcakes are made without any palm oil unlike most that are sold.

It's very difficult to buy oatcakes that are gluten-free, oil-free and wheat-free but easy to make your own. Freshly baked oatcakes taste much better than their shop bought counterparts.

Ingredients

- 1½ cups / 150g **Rolled oats**
- 2 tbsp **Sunflower seeds**
- 2 tbsp **Pumpkin seeds**
- 2 tbsp **Sesame seeds**
- 2 tbsp **Chia seeds**
- 2 tbsp **Flax seeds**
- a pinch **Salt**
- ¼ tsp **Baking soda**
- 1 cup / 235ml **Hot water**
- 2 tbsp Mixture of the **5 seeds**, to sprinkle on top

Equipment

- Small blender / coffee grinder
- Oven
- Greaseproof / parchment paper
- Bowl

Method

1. Pre-heat oven to 375F / 190C.
2. Grind the oats using a small blender. They don't have to be a fine powder, unless you want fine oatcakes. I like the rough type so 30 seconds is enough.
3. Mix together all the dry ingredients in a bowl and add the hot water a tablespoon at a time until it forms a solid dough that doesn't stick to your hands. Use boiled water that has been left to stand for a few minutes.
4. Form a firm ball with your hands. Add more oats if you've added too much water.
5. Leave the ball of dough to stand for 5 minutes to help it all stick together.
6. Press the dough out on non-stick paper using your fingers to form one piece about 5-10mm in thickness.
7. Sprinkle on a mix of 2 tbsp of all the seeds on top and press into the dough.
8. Bake for about 30 minutes until the oatcake starts to go golden.
9. Remove from the oven and cut into separate oatcakes while still hot.
10. Leave to cool for 10 minutes and then break apart and enjoy within 5 days, although they are best fresh.
11. Return to the oven for 5-10 minutes until bone dry if you want to store the oatcakes for several weeks.
12. Always store in an airtight container.

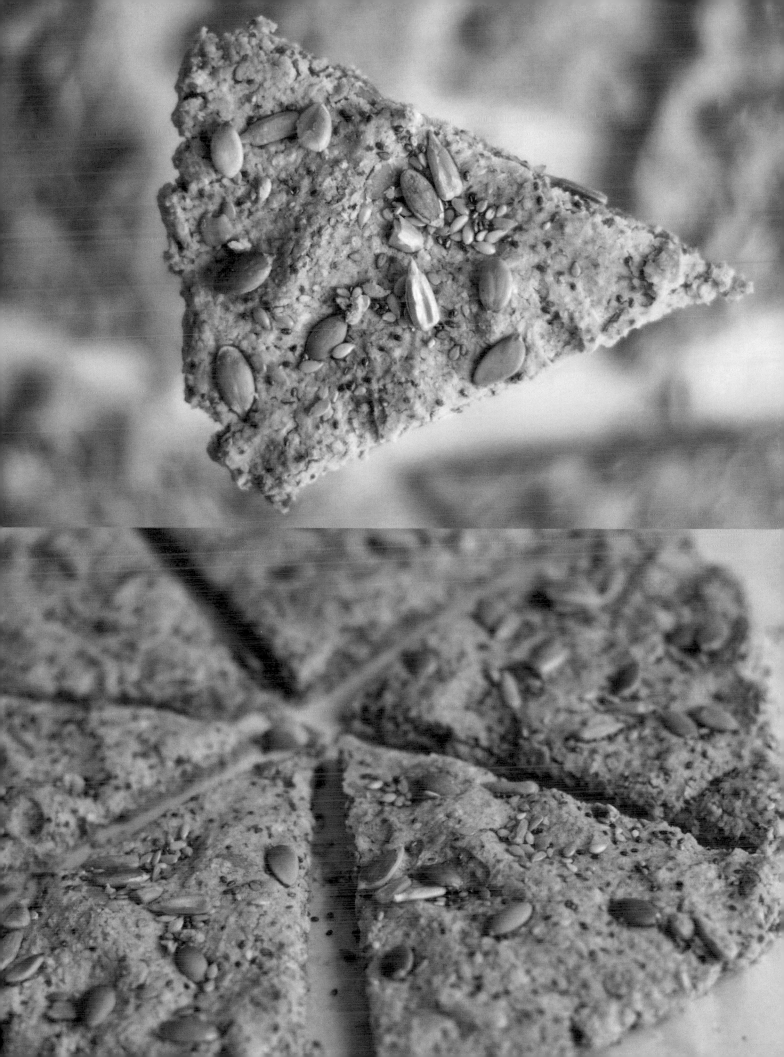

Avocado Mayo Sweet Potato Salad

Makes 10 servings | 10 mins **p**

Even organic vegan mayo mainly consists of unhealthy oil. This mayo is made of heart healthy fats from avocados and Brazil nuts and is a source of protein. It goes perfectly with steamed sweet potatoes to make a sweet potato salad that is a great side dish.

Avozil Mayo **raw**

- 2 medium **Avocados**
- 2 cloves **Garlic**
- 1 cup / 150g **Brazil nuts**
- 4 tbsp **Apple Cider Vinegar** (page 110)
- pinch of **Salt**

Sweet Potato Salad

- 1kg / 8 cups **Sweet potatoes**, pealed and diced. About 2 large, 3 medium or 6 small
- 2 handfuls **Cherry tomatoes**
- a few **Chives**

Equipment

- Blender and steamer

Mayo Method

1. Soak Brazil nuts in salted water for an hour or overnight.
2. Skin the avocados and garlic.
3. Place all in the blender with enough cider vinegar for the blender to do its job.
4. If it isn't blending add more apple cider vinegar / water depending on how vinegary you like it.

Sweet Potato Salad Method

5. Steam peeled diced sweet potatoes until cooked, about 20-25 minutes.
6. Mix together the cooked sweet potatoes and the mayo.
7. Sprinkle on the tomatoes, chives and paprika.
8. Store in the fridge and it will last for about 3 days.

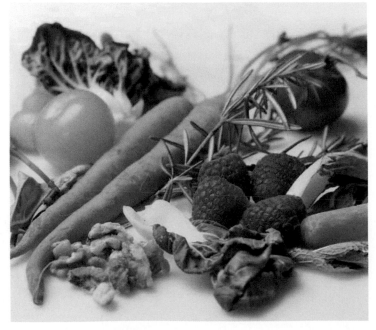

Natural Produce and Variation

All of the recipes in this book are high in natural produce. Unlike refined ingredients like flour and sugar these do vary significantly in flavour / sweetness / water content and other properties depending on the varieties, seasons and quality.

I'm always upset when a recipe didn't work out for someone but with plant-based recipes that are entirely natural produce, it's important to taste as you go and adjust as required.

Even the recipes that need cooking you can taste a tiny amount before cooking.

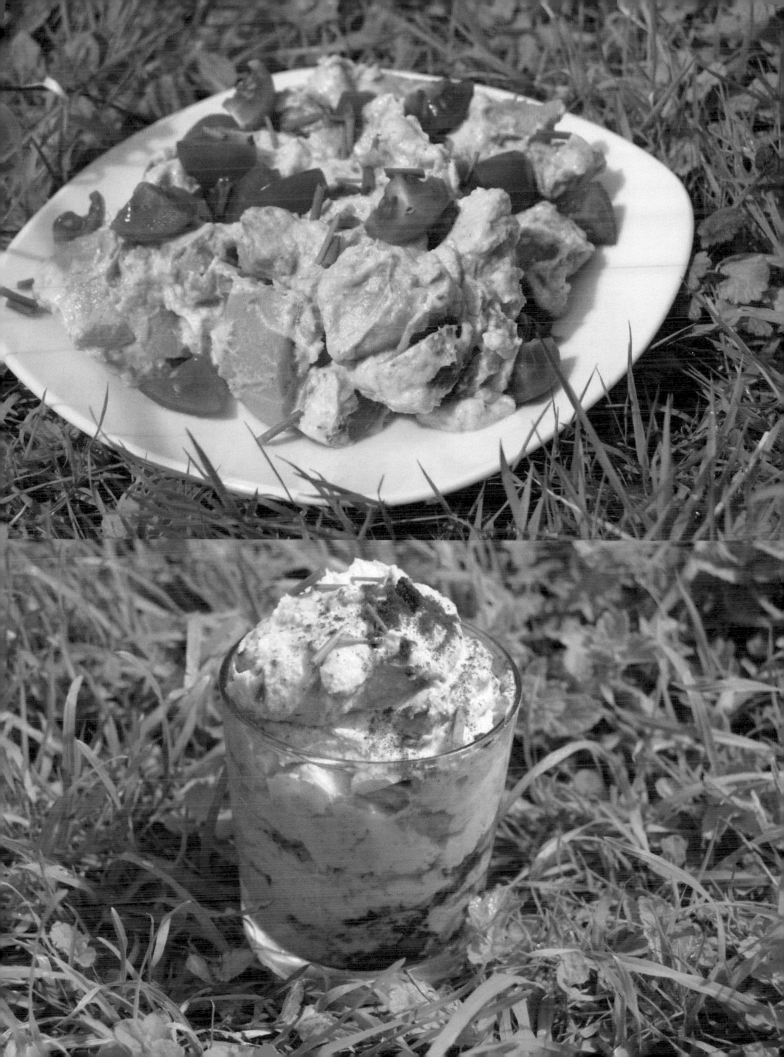

Sweet Potato Falafel With Sesame Lemon Dressing

Makes 9 falafels | 30 mins

This Sweet Potato Falafel is a delicious twist on a classic. The sweet potato, lemon zest and raisins give this falafel a unique taste and texture. You can eat in a wrap with salad or with tomatoes, pickles, ripped coriander and lashings of the sesame lemon dressing.

Falafel

- 1 can **Chickpeas**, 15oz / 400ml
- 2 tbsp grated **Sweet potato**
- 2 tbsp diced **Red onion**
- 2 cloves diced **Garlic**
- ½ juiced **Lemon** and 1" square rind chopped finely
- 1 tbsp **Tomato puree**
- 1 tbsp **Raisins**
- 1 tsp **Cumin**
- 1 tsp **Ground coriander**
- 1 tsp **Cayenne pepper**

Sesame Lemon Dressing

- 2 tbsp **Sesame seeds**, ground
- 1 tbsp **Olive oil**, optional
- 1 tsp **Garlic** clove
- 1 **Lemon**, juiced
- **Salt** and **Pepper** to taste
- a few **Coriander leaves** to garnish

Equipment

- Food processor
- Oven
- Tray
- Greaseproof paper

Method

1. Place all the falafel ingredients together in a blender and pulse for 30 seconds or so until broken up and combined.
2. Roll into about 9 balls of equal size.
3. Place on a non stick tray and bake at 390F / 200C for about 30 minutes until golden.
4. Turn half way through.
5. Mix together all the ingredients for the tahini lemon dressing.
6. Will last for a few days stored in the fridge. Drizzle on the dressing just before enjoying.

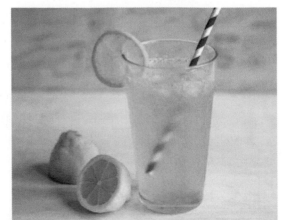

Lemon Zest

One of the stars of the show in this falafel is the lemon zest. It helps to give a slight bitter flavour that really elevates the dish. Try to get untreated and unwaxed lemons.

Bitter Lemon Tonic Water

Boil the rind of a lemon in a cup of water. Then cool and add to the juice of a lemon with a touch of sweetener and sparkling water for a refreshing slightly bitter tonic drink.

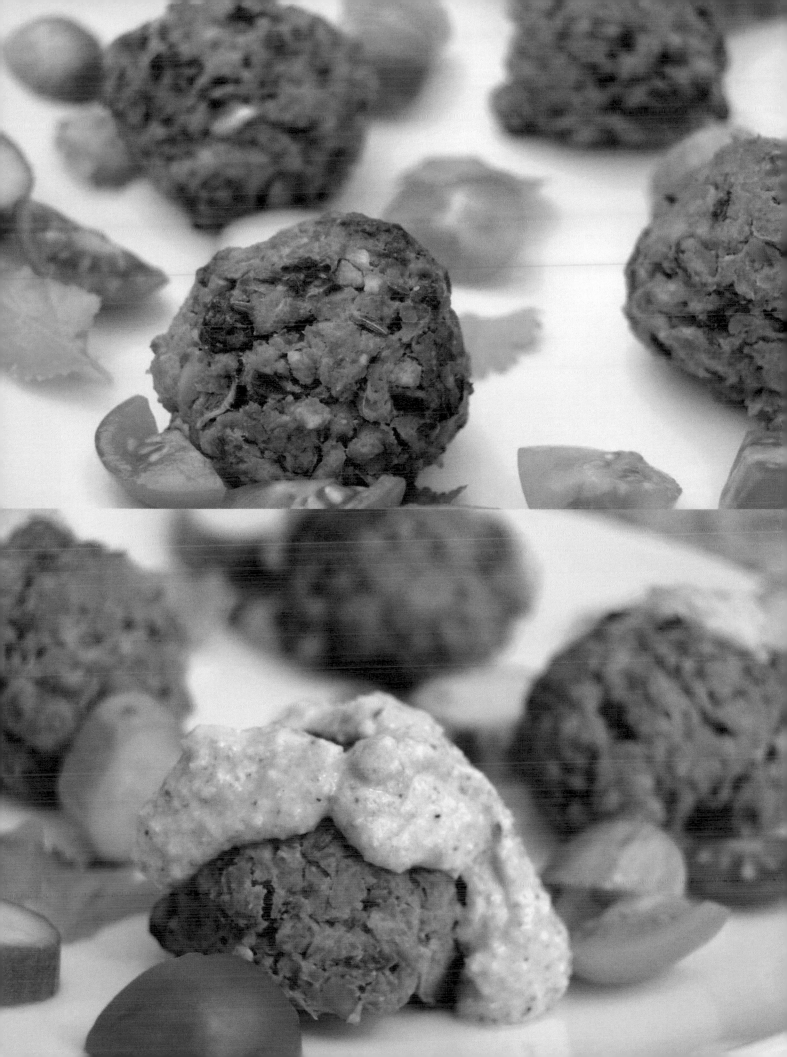

Beetroot and Bean Pots

Makes 2 pots | 5 mins **nf**

This high protein dip makes the perfect snack or light meal with raw veggies or your favourite bread. Perfect on the go food when placed in an airtight pot.

Ingredients

- 1 can **White beans / Cannelloni**, 15oz / 400ml
- 2 **Beetroot**, cooked
- 1 **Lemon**, juiced
- 1" square of **Lemon rind**
- 1 large **Garlic clove**
- 1 tbsp **Sesame seeds**
- ¼ tsp **Cayenne pepper**
- ½ tsp **Cumin**
- pinch of **Salt** and **Pepper**
- a handful of **Rocket**
- 2 tbsp **Broad beans**, frozen thawed

Equipment

- Blender and Pots

Method

1. Place everything in a food processor apart from the rocket and broad beans,
2. Blend until smooth and all broken up.
3. Spoon into pots.
4. Top with rocket and broad beans.
5. Keep chilled and eat within 3 days.

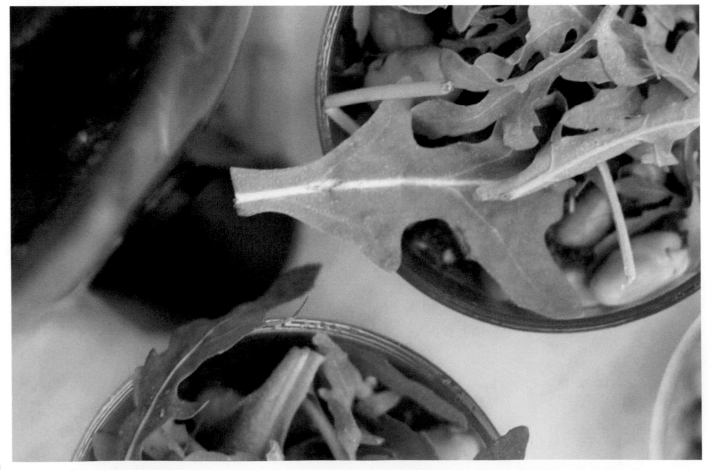

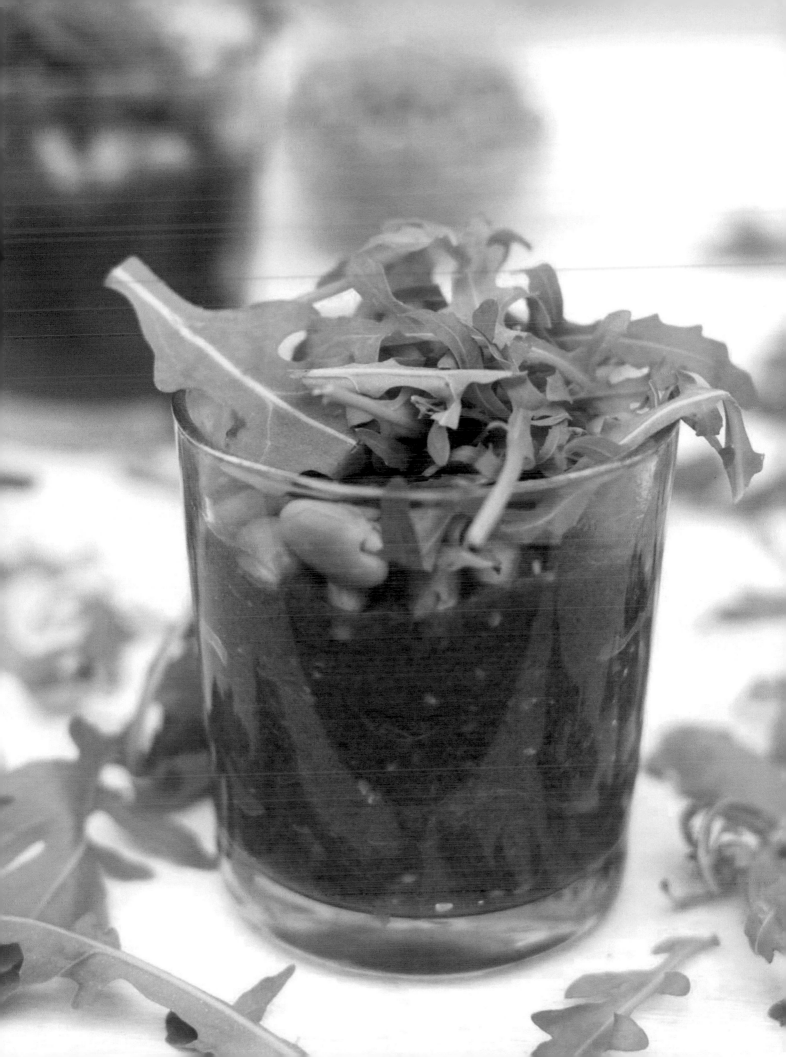

Cashew Mozzarella Quinoa Pizza

Makes 6 slices | 1h

Easy quinoa crust pizza that is topped with melted cashew mozzarella. It may look like a lot of ingredients and take an hour in total to make but each step is easy. The oven is doing all work and only a small amount of prep is needed.

The cashew mozzarella is especially quick and easy to make - the only way you can really go wrong is not stirring enough and the bottom burning.

Quinoa Crust

- ¾ cup / 135g **Quinoa**
- ½ tsp **Cayenne pepper**
- ½ tsp **Baking powder**
- ¾ cup / 175ml **Water**
- ¼ tsp **Salt**

Pizza Topping Ingredients

Use any that you like, this is just a guide:

- 4 tbsp **Sieved tomatoes** / tomato paste
- handful of **Basil leaves**

Cashew Mozzarella Cheese

- ⅓ cup / 50g **Cashews**
- 2 tbsp **Nutritional Yeast** (page 108)
- 1 clove **Garlic**
- 1 cup / 240ml **Water**
- pinch of **Salt**
- 2 tbsp **Tapioca Starch** (page 170)

Equipment

- Pan & Oven
- Greaseproof / parchment paper

Method

1. Soak the quinoa for 15 minutes or overnight.
2. Rinse and drain the quinoa then put in a blender jug with all the other crust ingredients and blend until smooth.
3. Line an 8" pan with greaseproof paper or just use a silicon pan and pour in the quinoa batter.
4. Bake for 30-35 minutes at 375F / 190C, until a knife comes out clean. Let stand for 5 minutes and then take out of the pan.
5. Bake for 10 minutes with no tray at 375F / 190C, just to make it crispy on both sides.
6. Put all of the cashew mozzarella ingredients apart from the tapioca starch into a blender and blend until smooth.
7. Empty the mozzarella mixture into a pan and sift in the tapioca starch.
8. Heat gently while stirring constantly to stop the bottom from burning. It's ready when its thick and gooey and rolls off the spoon slowly.
9. Spread the tomato passata over the base, then blob on the cashew mozzarella and sprinkle with basil leaves.

Notes

You can place back into the oven to brown up the cashew cheese. I didn't here as the base straight out of the oven and the cheese just off the pan was already hot enough for me.

The small picture to the right shows how stringy the cheese for this pizza is.

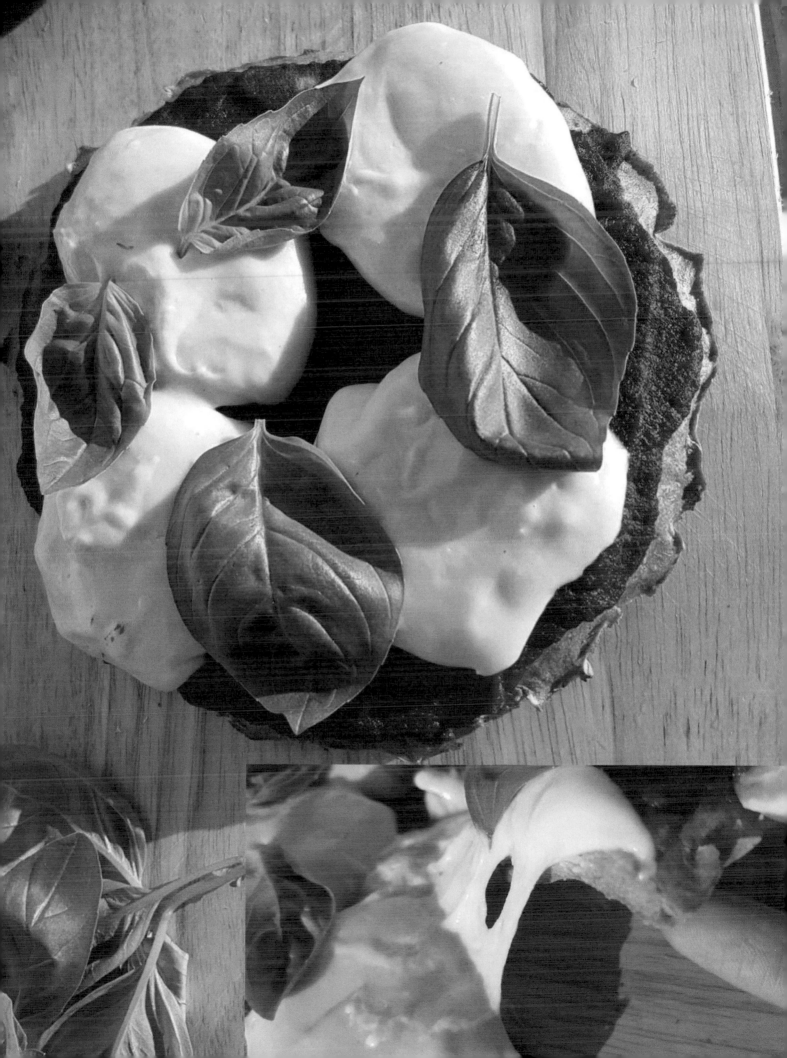

Cheesy Protein Pasta

Serves 2 | 15 mins **nf**

This healthy cheesy protein pasta is vegan and gluten free. One serving contains 41 grams of protein. It's also high in calcium from the sesame seeds and beans.

As nutritional yeast contains all nine essential ammo acids it provides a complete plant protein.

Ingredients

- 1 can **White beans**, 15oz / 400g
- 2½ cups / 160g **Bean / Lentil Pasta**
- 4 tbsp **Nutritional Yeast** (page 108)
- ½ cup / 120ml **Water**
- 1 **Garlic** clove
- 2 tbsp **Sesame seeds**
- ¼ tsp **Turmeric**
- 1 tbsp **Apple Cider Vinegar** (page 110)
- ½ tsp **Smoked paprika**
- ½ tsp **Chopped basil**
- pinch of **Salt** and **Pepper**

Equipment

- Blender
- Pan

Method

1. Place everything apart from the pasta into a blender and whizz until combined.
2. Cook the pasta as per instructions and drain.
3. Stir in the cheesy bean pasta sauce.
4. Serve with smoked paprika and basil sprinkled on top.
5. Store leftovers in the fridge and enjoy within three days.

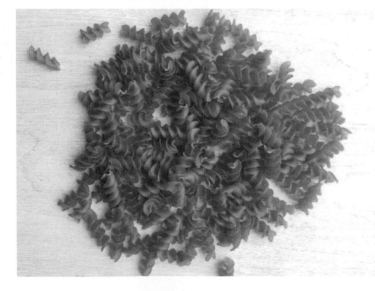

Bean and Lentil Pasta

There are many different types of gluten-free pasta that are made from 100% beans or lentils.

I'm using red lentil fusilli for this recipe as it's wildly available in normal food shops and has a similar taste and texture to normal pasta. It starts off a bright red but loses this colour after being cooked. Other bean pastas I recommend are mung bean fettuccine and black bean spaghetti.

Bean Cheese Sauce

For a velvety creamy dairy-free cheese style sauce use the basic recipe here of beans, nutritional yeast, garlic and sesame seeds.

You can use any white beans for this like cannellini, navy or butter. Replace the sesame with nuts or sunflower seeds if you prefer.

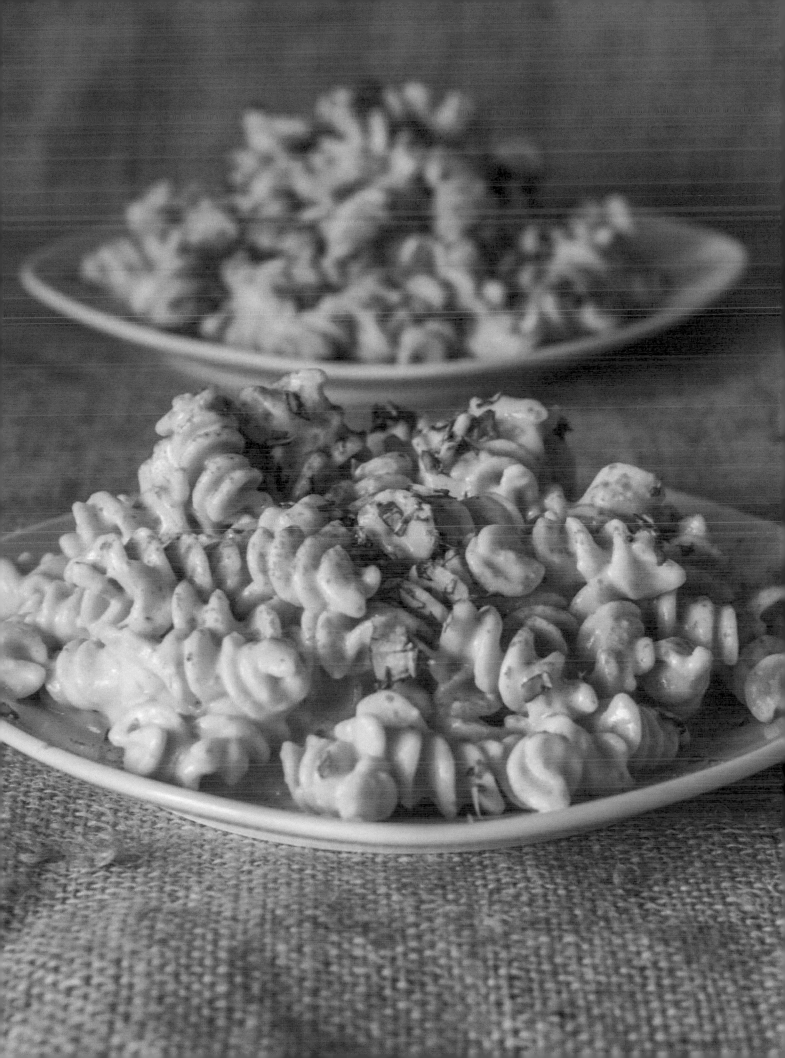

Quinoa Vegetable Seed Sliders

Makes 9 sliders | 1h 15 mins **nf**

These quinoa flatbread sliders may look like a lot of ingredients, but the recipe is as simple as blending and baking. They are very filling and bursting with nutrition. This could easily serve 4 as a main meal as they are so satisfying and a complete meal full of protein and carbohydrates.

Quinoa Flatbread

- 2 cups **Quinoa**
- 2 **Garlic cloves**
- ¼ tsp **Turmeric**
- ¼ tsp **Cayenne pepper**
- ¼ tsp **Baking powder**
- 3 tbsp **Chia** seeds, soaked 9 tbsp **Water**
- 1 cup / 240ml **Water**
- pinch of **Salt** and **Pepper**
- **Water** for soaking

Sundried Tomato Ketchup

- 8 **Sun-dried** tomatoes, soaked
- 4 tbsp **Apple Cider Vinegar** (page 110)

Fillings and Topping

- 8 **Gherkins**, sliced lengthways
- handful of **Rocket**
- 2 tbsp **Sesame seeds**

Seed and Vegetable Burgers

- ½ cup **Sunflower seed**
- ½ cup **Pumpkin seeds**
- 1 **Carrot**
- 1 **Celery stick**
- 1 small **Red onion**
- 1 heaped tsp **Smoked paprika**
- pinch of **Salt** and **Pepper**
- 3 tbsp ground **Chia** seeds, soaked 9 tbsp **Water**
- **Water** for soaking

Equipment

- Blender
- Food processor
- Oven
- 2 Square 8" baking dishes
- Greaseproof paper

Method

1. Soak the quinoa in one bowl and the sunflower and pumpkin seeds in another with water and a pinch of salt. 8 hours soaking time is ideal but an hour is sufficient.
2. Drain the quinoa and add to a blender with all the other flatbread ingredients.
3. Blend until smooth and then pour into a greaseproof paper lined tray about 8" square.
4. Drain the pumpkin and sunflower seeds then add to a food processor along with everything else for the burgers.
5. Blend until combined and sticking together. Spread out in a lined tray about 8" square.
6. Bake both at 375F / 190C for 50-60 minutes until a knife comes out clean.
7. Leave to cool and firm up while blending the tomatoes and vinegar for the ketchup.
8. Turn out the flatbread and slice in half horizontally.
9. Place the burger on the flatbread, spread over a layer of ketchup, sliced gherkins, rocket then put on the flatbread top.
10. Cut into 12 squares, sprinkle on sesame seeds and enjoy within 3 days.

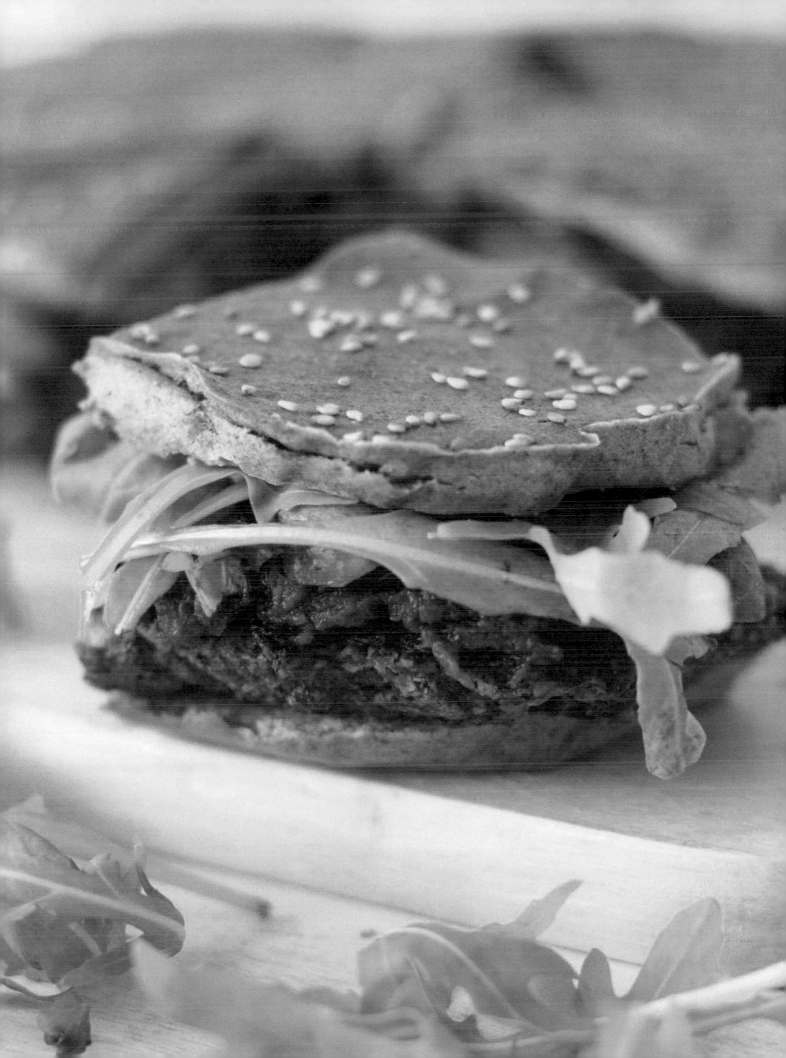

Crushed Chickpea Hummus Salad

Single main serving | Serves 4 as a side | 20 mins **nf**

Quick easy homemade hummus topped with basil, red onion, black olives, tomatoes, cucumber, and avocado. This recipe is simple but full of flavoursome fresh fruit and vegetables that give it a strong taste.

This is one of my all time favourite dishes to make as it's satisfying, tasty, easily made and bursting with nutrition.

Hummus

- 1 can **Chickpeas**, 15oz / 400ml
- 1 **Lemon**, juiced
- 2 tbsp **Sesame seeds**, ground
- 2 cloves **Garlic**, crushed
- ¼ tsp **Cayenne pepper**
- ¼ tsp **Turmeric**
- ¼ tsp **Cumin**
- **Salt** & **Pepper**, to taste

Mediterranean Salad

- 16 **Basil** leaves
- 10 **Cherry tomatoes**, quartered
- 2" **Cucumber,** diced
- ½ **Avocado**, diced
- 10 **Black olives**, halved
- 1 slice **Red onion**, diced
- 1 tsp dried **Thyme**
- 2 tbsp **Olive oil**, optional

Method

1. Drain and rinse the chickpeas.
2. Mash the chickpeas using the back of a fork or a potato masher.
3. Grind the sesame seeds in a small jug or coffee blender.
4. Mix all of the hummus ingredients with the chickpeas.
5. Spread the hummus into a bowl making a well to fill with the basil leaves and the other fruit and vegetables.
6. Sprinkle with dried thyme and drizzle with olive oil.
7. Store in the fridge and enjoy within 2 days.

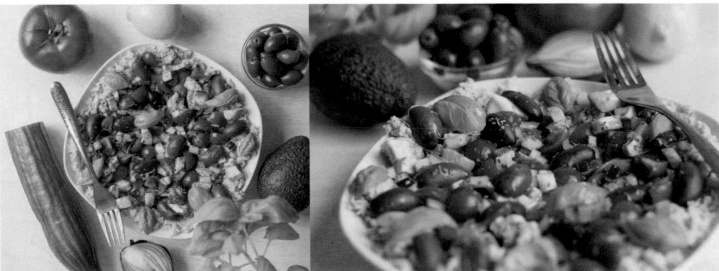

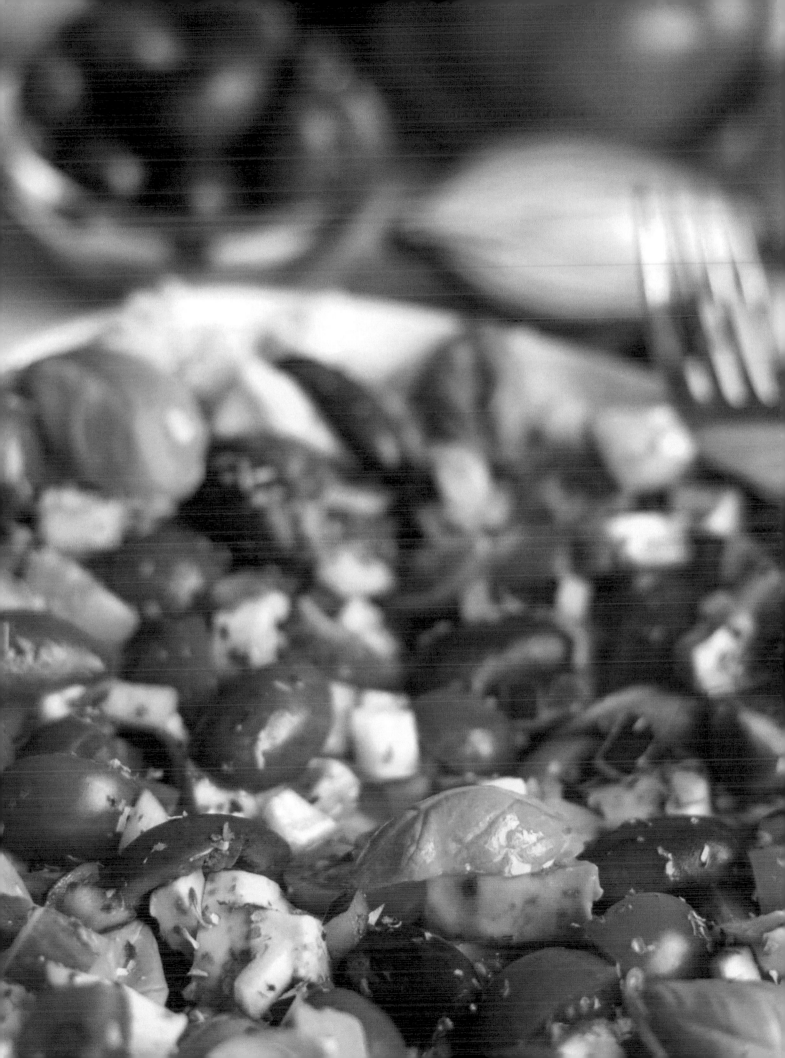

Avocado on Quinoa Bread Toast

Serves 4 | 1h **nf**

This avocado quinoa toast is easy to make and naturally gluten free. Top with smashed avocado for amazing gluten-free avocado toast. The quinoa flatbread has a nutty flavour that is far tastier than normal bread. The base may take a bit of time with soaking and baking, but little prep is needed. So while it isn't quick it's still very easy to make.

Quinoa Flatbread

- ¾ cup / 135g **Quinoa**
- ½ tsp **Cayenne Pepper**
- ½ tsp **Baking Powder**
- pinch of **Salt**
- ¾ cup / 175ml **Water**

Topping Suggestions

- 1 **Avocado**
- slice of **Red Onion**
- **Cherry Tomatoes & Cress**

Equipment

- **Oven, Baking pan** & **Greaseproof paper**

Method

1. Soak the quinoa for 15 minutes or more in water.
2. Rinse and drain the quinoa then put in a blender jug with all the other flatbread ingredients and blend until smooth.
3. Line a 8" pan with greaseproof paper or just use a silicon pan and pour in the quinoa batter.
4. Bake for 20 minutes at 450F / 230C, take out of the pan and then bake for 10 more minutes.
5. Let the flat bread cool and then cover with the smashed avocado and other toppings.

Notes

Most quinoa for sale in the US and UK is pre-rinsed so doesn't need to be rinsed well after soaking. But if yours has a bitter taste this usually suggests that it hasn't been rinsed and needs a good thorough rinse after being soaked.

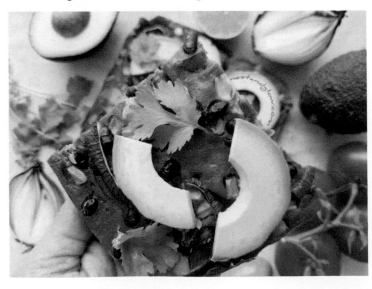

Mexican Quinoa Flatbread

This variation has a tomato quinoa base with beans and corn baked in. Topped with creamy avocado, zesty lime juice and fragrant coriander.

Adapt the original by adding 4 tbsp **Tomato puree** to the base blended mixture. Then sprinkle on about 2tbsp of **Corn, Black beans** and **Red onion** just before baking. Once baked garnish with **Avocado, Coriander** and **Lime** juice.

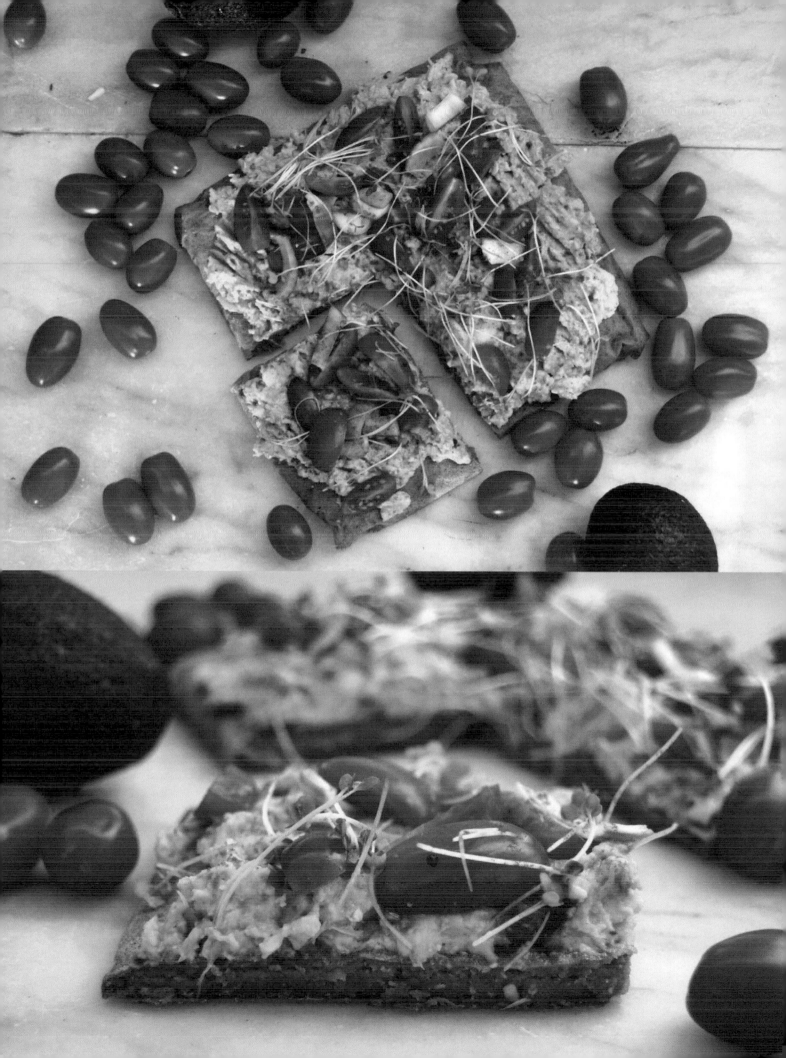

Rainbow Noodles with Parmesan

Serves 4 | 1h

These colourful noodles are very easy to make and completely natural. You can use this recipe to dye any kind of pasta or noodles a bright vibrant colour without any e-numbers or anything artificial in sight.

The parmesan is made without using any machines and is a useful condiment for sprinkling onto savoury dishes. I often make in bulk to have a large pre-mixed jar in the cupboard.

Ingredients

- 8.8 oz / 250g uncooked **Noodles** or **Pasta**, I used gluten free rice noodles

Yellow natural dye

- 1 tbsp **Turmeric**
- 1 cup / 250ml **Water**

Purple natural dye

- ⅕ **Red cabbage**, juiced
- a few tbsp of **Water** to help blend

Blue natural dye

- ⅕ **Red cabbage**, juiced
- pinch of **Baking soda**

Red natural dye

- **Beetroot**, cooking juice

Green natural dye

- Mix together 50 / 50 Blue and Yellow dye

Vegan parmesan

- 3 tbsp ground **Almonds**
- 2 tbsp **Nutritional Yeast** (page 108)
- 1 tsp **Garlic powder**
- a pinch of **Salt**
- 1 tbsp **cold pressed Oil**, optional but helps to combine

Equipment

- Pan and 5 bowls

Method

1. Juice the red cabbage and then separate into two bowls. One will be your purple dye and to the other add baking soda to make blue.
2. Boil 1 tbsp turmeric with 1 cup / 250 ml water for 2 minutes. Strain and you have your yellow dye.
3. For red either boil beetroot for a few minutes in water and use this water or just drain off the juice from pre-cooked vacuum packed beetroot (without vinegar).
4. Mix together half of the yellow and blue (50 / 50) to make green.
5. Cook the noodles / pasta that you are using until they are al dente so still have a bit of a bite, they will soften when soaked in the dye.
6. Then separate the noodles/pasta into 5 bowls.
7. Mix 4-6 tbsp of the natural food dyes with the noodles and leave to colour for 20 minutes. Stir half way through.
8. Mix all the ingredients for the vegan parmesan in a bowl.
9. Drain the noodles from the dye and then mix all the noodles and sprinkle with the vegan parmesan.
10. You can enjoy these cold or just put in the oven or microwave for a few minutes to heat up.

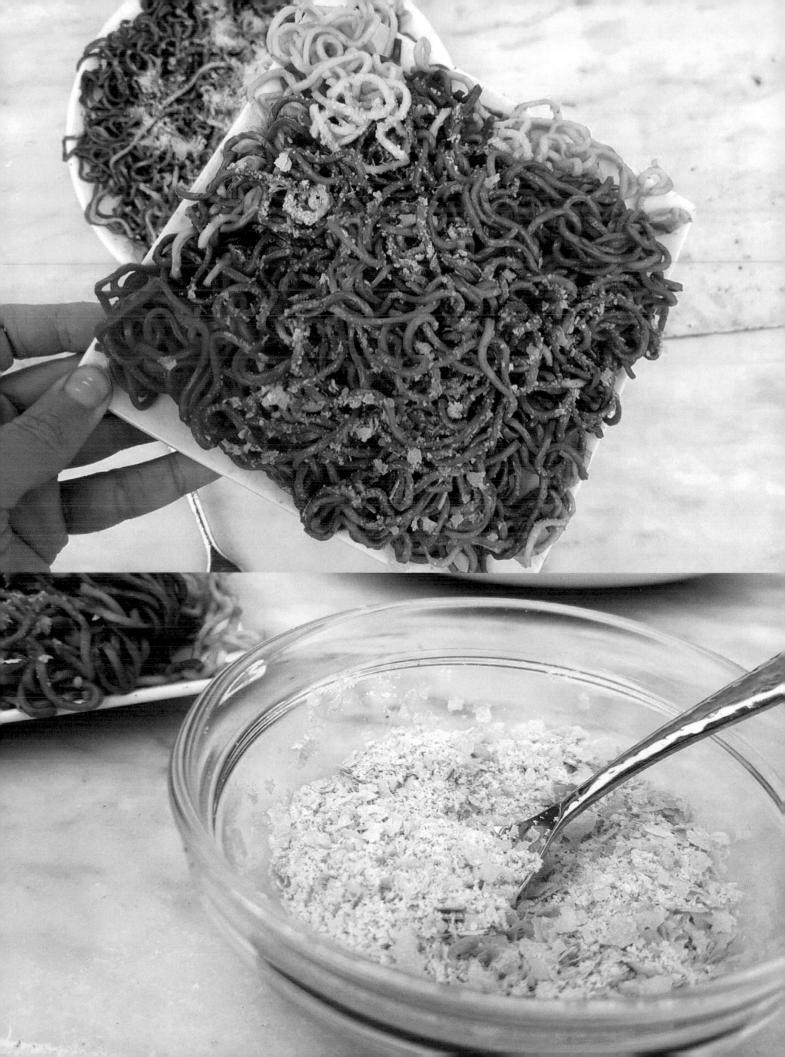

Sunflower Cheese Raw Courgetti

Serves 2 | 20 mins (raw) (p) (nf)

This quick and easy recipe for sunflower seed cheesy spaghetti uses courgette (zucchini) to make courgetti. The creamy seed-based sauce makes a filling low-carb and dairy-free meal. Instead of cooking, the courgettes are massaged with salt to give a soft cooked like texture without cooking out any of the goodness.

Ingredients

- 1 cup / 140g **Sunflower seeds**
- 3 **Courgette/Zucchini**
- 3 tbsp **Nutritional Yeast** (page 108)
- 1 **Garlic clove**
- 3 tbsp **Sesame seeds**
- **Basil leaves**
- ¼ tsp **Turmeric**
- 1 tbsp **Apple Cider Vinegar** (page 110)
- 6 **Cherry tomatoes**
- 2 pinches of **Salt**
- **Water** for soaking and blending

Equipment

- Blender and Spiralizer

Method

1. Soak the sunflower seeds in a pinch of salt for an hour or overnight.
2. Drain the sunflower seed and then add to a blender with the nutritional yeast, garlic, sesame, vinegar and turmeric.
3. Add just enough water to help your blender whizz into a smooth paste.
4. Spiralize your courgette/zucchini using a spiralizer. If you don't have one try a julienne slicer or vegetable peeler to make thin strips.
5. Massage a pinch of salt into the courgette until it goes down in volume by about a third and releases it's juices.
6. Stir in the sunflower seed cheese and enjoy.
7. Store any left-overs in the fridge and eat within 48 hours.

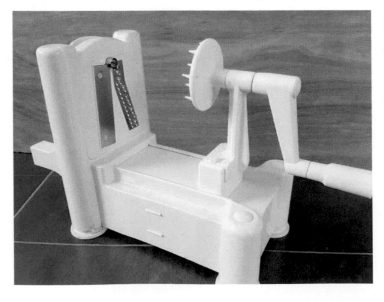

Spiralizer

These gadgets turn vegetables or fruit into oodles of noodles very quickly. They work really well with courgettes, carrots, beetroot, sweet potato, apple and cucumbers to name a few.

Spiralizers often have several different attachments to create either thin noddles, thick noodles or ribbons.

Incredibly useful to make gluten-free low carb alternatives to pasta products. Also very helpful to make fresh produce more appetising.

154

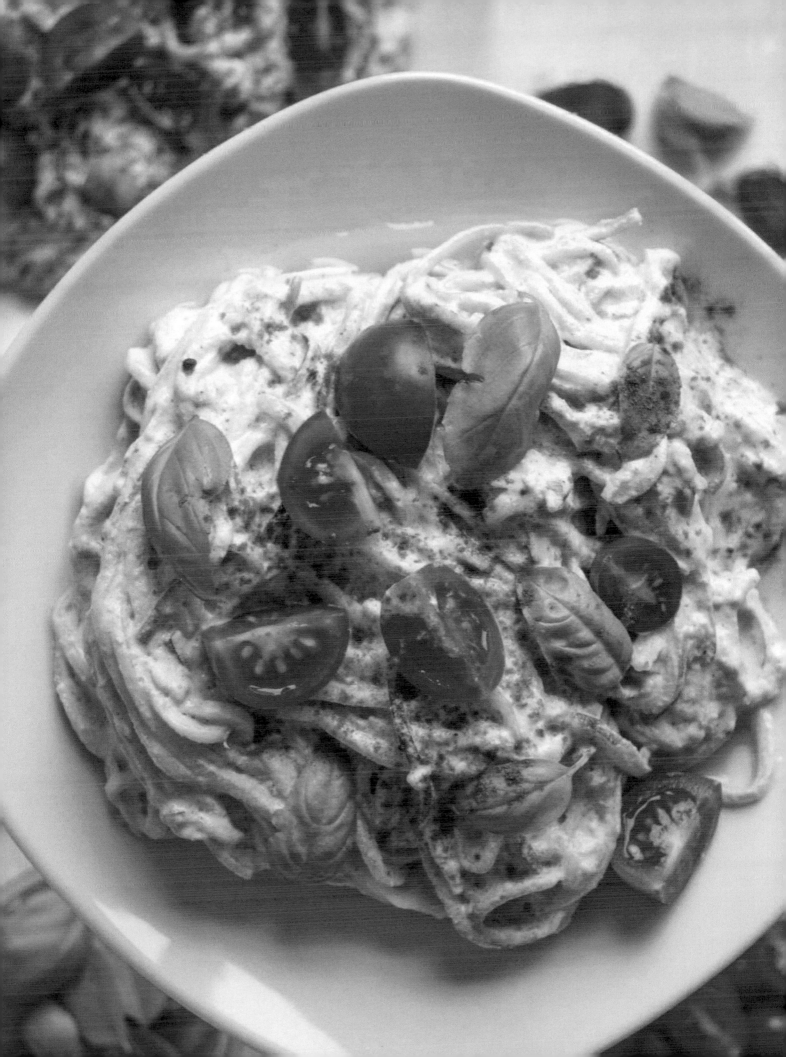

Soured Chickpea Lemon Curry

Serves 2 | 20 mins **nf**

Although the name of this recipe is soured chickpeas they aren't actually sour as the natural sweetness of the tomatoes and onion balances the dish. Lemon juice gives the sour flavour and the sweetness from the tomatoes, the spiciness from the chilli and the saltiness all together give a great depth of flavour.

The dish is finished with raw lemon juice, onion, garlic and chilli to give a mixture of flavours and textures.

Ingredients

- 2 **Onions**, diced
- 5 cloves of **Garlic**, diced
- 1 can chopped **Tomatoes**, 15oz / 400ml
- 1 can **Chickpeas**, 15oz / 400ml
- 1 tsp **Garam masala**
- ½ tsp ground **Cumin**
- ½ tsp **Turmeric**
- ½ tsp **Cayenne pepper**
- 2 **Lemons**, juiced
- 1" **Ginger**, pealed and diced
- fresh **Chilli pepper**, to taste
- **Salt**, a pinch
- 1 tbsp chopped **Coriander**

Method

1. Fry the onions and garlic for 4-5 minutes until softened. I "fry" in a few tbsp of water for health reasons but use oil if you prefer.
2. Add the tomatoes, chickpeas and ground spices and simmer for 10 minutes with the lid on, stirring occasionally.
3. Juice the lemons and mix with the diced ginger, a diced clove of garlic and the chilli finely ground. Let it mingle for 5 minutes while the curry cooks.
4. Stir in the sour lemon mixture and serve with shredded coriander.

Garam Masala

This is a mix of different spices usually containing pepper, cloves, cinnamon, mace, cardamom, bay leaf, cumin and coriander. However the ingredients do vary significantly depending on the region. The word garam means hot and these spices are believed to "heat the body."

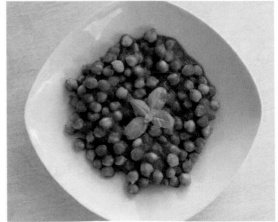

2 Minute Chickpea Curry

This single serving curry is almost too basic to list as a recipe but I eat it regularly. The ingredients are always in my cupboard as they are not fresh, but it still makes a nutritious meal.

Drain 1 tin of **Chickpeas** into a pan, add a couple of tbsp of **Water** and turn on to a high heat. Add 4 tbsp **Tomato puree**, ½ tsp of **Cumin**, **Turmeric**, **Cayenne** & **Onion powder** while constantly stirring for 2 minutes in total.

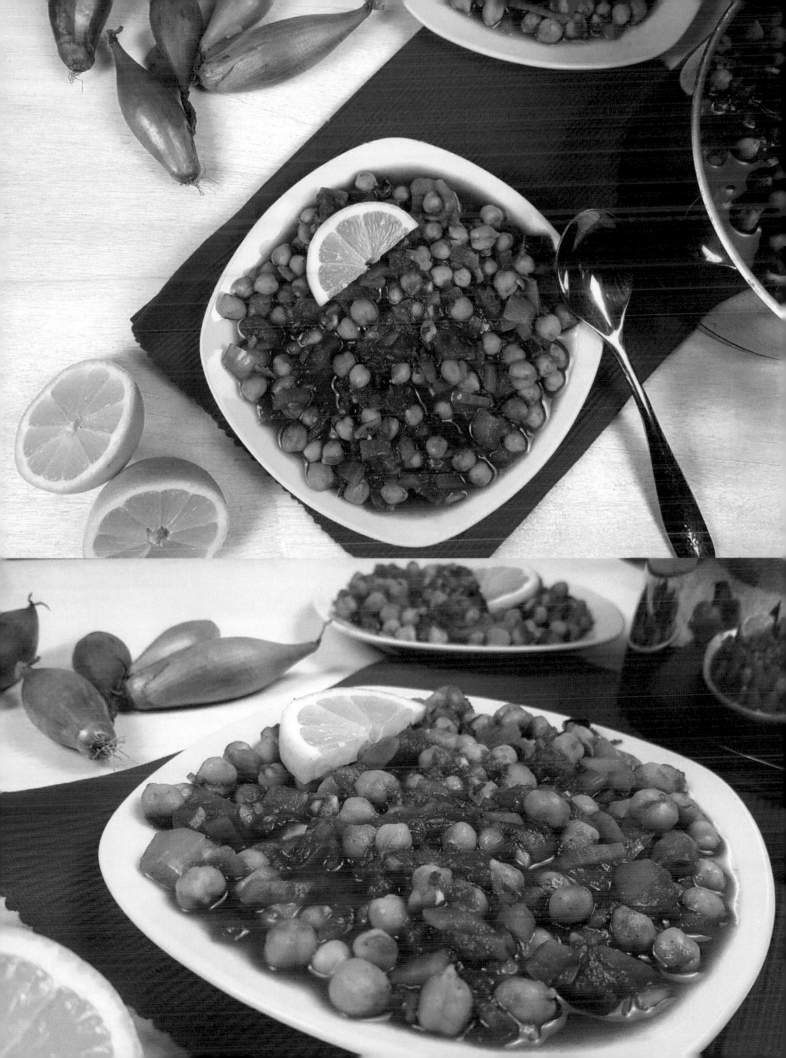

One-pot Tomato Basil Quinoa

Serves 4 | 25 mins

This one pot quinoa recipe could not be simpler to make and is full of taste. It takes about 20 minutes to cook but you can just let it bubble away unwatched while you get on with something else.

As quinoa is a seed this is grain and gluten free so a perfect high carbohydrate alternative to pasta and rice. Quinoa contains all of the essential amino acids and is high in protein.

Ingredients

- 1 ¾ cups / 300g **Quinoa**
- 3 cups / 450g **Cherry tomatoes**, quartered
- 4 cups / 1 litre **Water**
- 1 large **Onion**, thinly sliced
- 4 cloves of **Garlic**, thinly sliced
- 2 springs of **Basil**
- 1 tbsp **Seaweed**
- 1 tbsp **Italian herbs**
- ½ tsp **Cayenne pepper**
- a pinch of **Black pepper**
- Olives, Nutritional yeast and Basil to top

Equipment

- Pan

Method

1. Place everything in a pan and bring to a boil.
2. Reduce to a simmer, cover and cook for 15-20 minutes until soft and fluffy.
3. Stir half way through. Fluff the quinoa with a fork and serve with the garnishes.
4. Store any leftovers in the fridge and enjoy within three days.

Notes

I often cook this in a pressure cooker as you can get beautiful fluffy quinoa when cooked for 6-7 minutes on the medium pressure setting.

You could fry the onion in oil if you like, but for health reasons nothing is fried in this book.

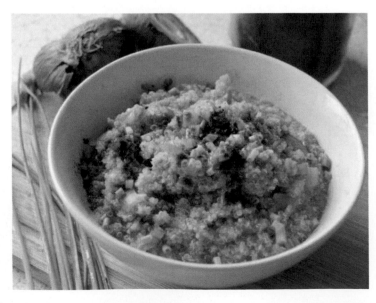

Curried Quinoa

Make a golden turmeric one pot curried quinoa with the same method as above but with the following ingredients:

- 1 ¾ cups / 300g **Quinoa**
- 1 large **Onion**, thinly sliced
- 4 cloves of **Garlic**, thinly sliced
- 1 tbsp **Turmeric**
- 1 tsp **Cayenne pepper** or **curry powder**
- 1 tsp **Cumin**
- serve with **Chives, Hot Paprika** & **Olive oil**

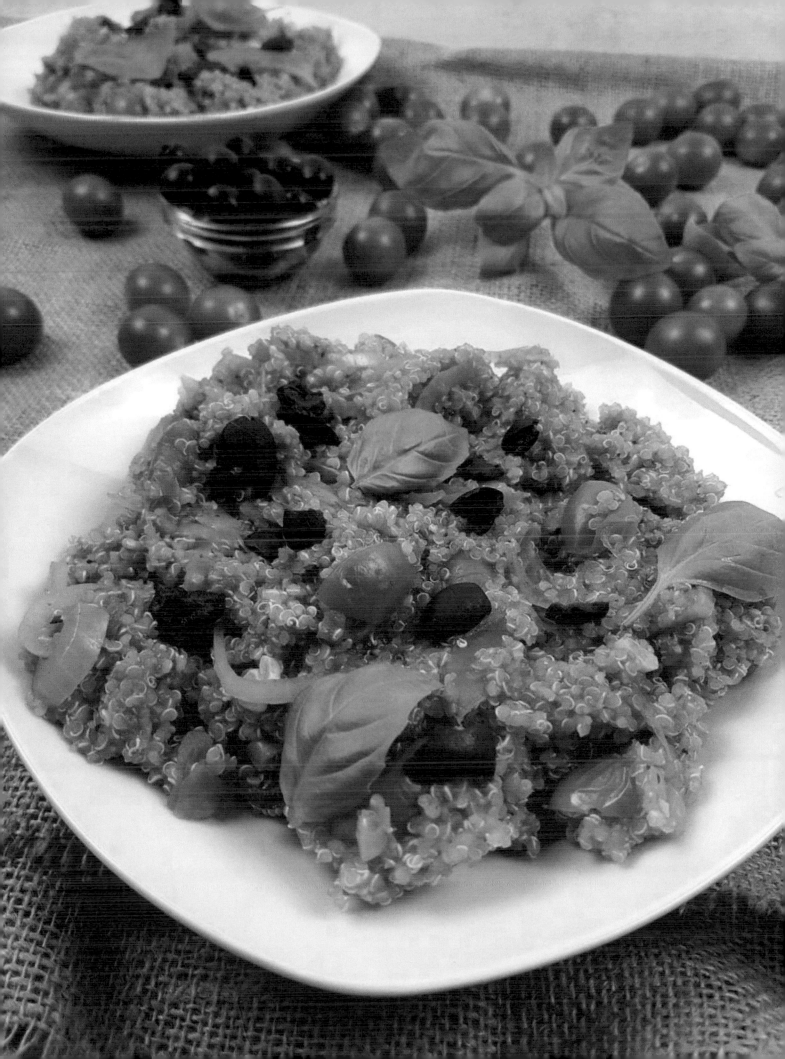

Chickpea Scrambled Eggs

Single serving | 30 mins **nf**

This high protein vegan scrambled chickpea "eggs" has a similar taste and texture to normal scrambled eggs. It's easy and cheap to make using home made chickpea tofu. Don't be put off if you don't like normal tofu as this soy-free chickpea version is very different.

Ingredients

- ½ cup / 65g **Chickpea flour**
- 1½ cups / 350ml **Water**
- ¼ tsp **Turmeric**
- ½ tsp **Smoked paprika**
- 1 clove **Garlic**
- 1 slice **Red onion**
- 3 tbsp **Vegetable broth**
- ½ tsp **Kala Namak / Black Salt**

Equipment

- Pan
- Bowl

Chickpea Tofu

Steps 1-5 of this recipe makes chickpea tofu. Buy your chickpea flour in a bulk from an Asian shop for the best price.

Perfect on veggie kebabs or in place of normal tofu.

Method

1. Mix together the chickpea flour, turmeric and smoked paprika with a third of the water into a paste.
2. Bring the other 2/3rd of the water to a simmer with a pinch of salt.
3. Stir in the chickpea mixture into the water and stir constantly for 5 minutes while simmering.
4. Be careful not to let the bottom of the mixture catch.
5. Remove from the heat and pour into a glass dish.
6. Chill for half an hour in the fridge then it should come away easily from the dish.
7. Mash the chickpea tofu in a pan and then add the remaining ingredients.
8. Cook for a few minutes until all the broth is absorbed and serve.
9. You can store the chickpea tofu in the fridge for a few days before cooking.

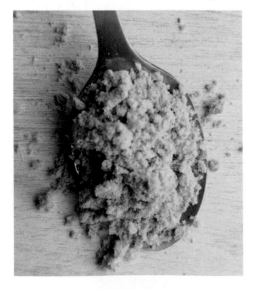

Kala Namak / Black Salt

Kala Namak is otherwise known as Himalayan Black Salt and is a natural rock salt. Black salt is a common ingredient in many Asian cuisines and can be found at even small Asian shops. It has an eggy taste due to the high sulphur content.

In large chunks the salt is black but once it's ground into a fine powder it goes a light purple / pink colour. You can use in place of normal salt to give an eggy taste in recipes such as avocado on toast. Western health food shops are now starting to stock it but the same product can be acquired significantly cheaper at most Asian supermarkets.

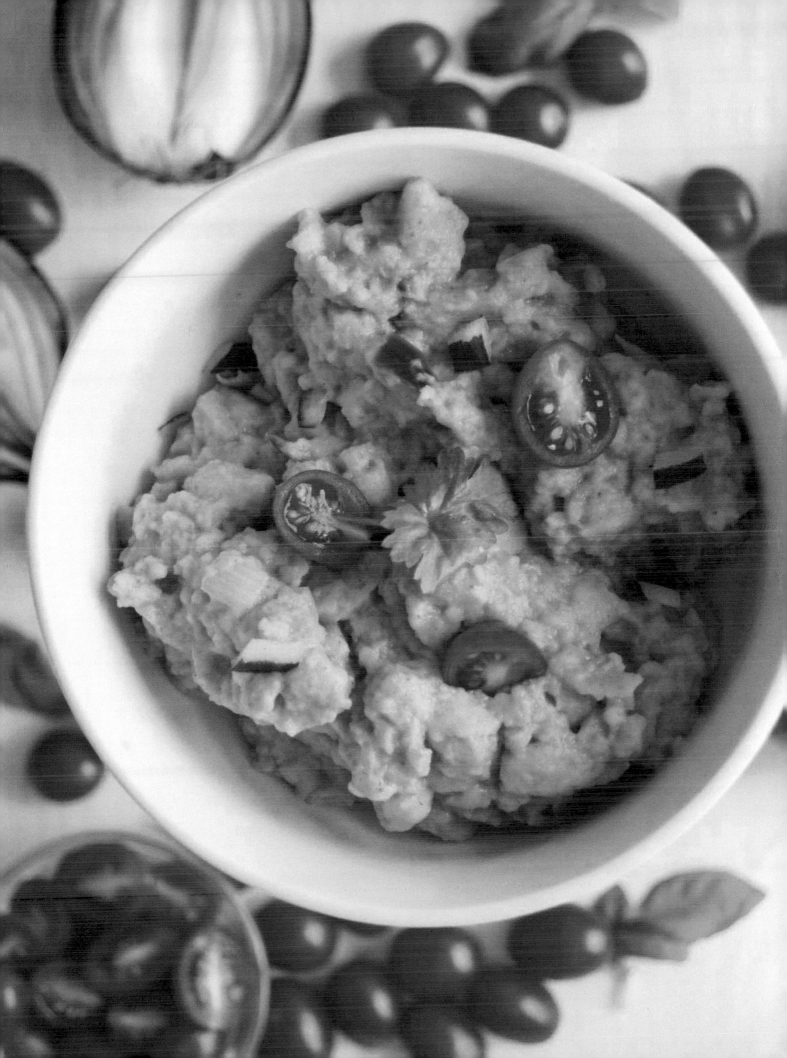

Tex-Mex Loaded Sweet Potato Skins

Serves 4 as sides | 1h 10 mins **nf**

These Tex-Mex Loaded Sweet Potato Skins are a real crowd-pleaser. A delicious complete meal full of protein and carbohydrates that is easy to make. It takes over an hour to do this recipe, but 90% of this is the oven baking the potatoes while you sit back and relax.

Ingredients

- 6 medium **Sweet potatoes**
- 1 cup / 200g **Black beans**
- 1 cup / 160g **Sweetcorn**, precooked
- 1 **Chilli**, de-seeded
- slice of **Onion**
- 1 cup / 150g **Cherry tomatoes**
- 1 bunch of **Coriander** / cilantro
- 1 tsp **Garlic**
- 1 **Lime**
- 2 **Avocados**

Equipment

- Oven and Tray

Sweet Potatoes and Yams

In north America what most people call a "yam" is actually a sweet potato. A real yam is a white starchy root that has scaly skin similar to tree bark.

It's now a legal requirement in the US for any label with yam to also have sweet potato but many still call sweet potatoes yams.

Method

1. Cut the ends off each sweet potato and then cut into half.
2. Place skin side down on a baking sheet and bake in the oven for about an hour at 400°F / 200°C until soft.
3. Remove from the oven and leave to cool for a few minutes.
4. Scoop out the insides of the sweet potatoes, being careful to not rip through the skin.
5. Put the sweet potato skins back in the oven at 200°F / 100°C to crisp up, but not burn, while you make the filling.
6. Mix together the sweet potato flesh with the black beans, sweet corn, sliced chilli, quartered cherry tomatoes, roughly chopped coriander / cilantro, minced garlic and the juice of the limes.
7. Take the skins out of the oven and pile on the filling as high as you can.
8. Top with cubes of avocado and enjoy!

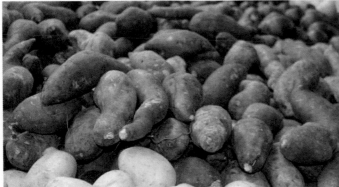

Sweet Potatoes Vs Normal Potatoes

You may notice that this book contains many sweet potato recipes and only one white potato recipe. While they both contain vitamins and minerals sweet potatoes are more nutrient dense. Despite having more sugar they are lower in over-all carbohydrates and lower in GI.

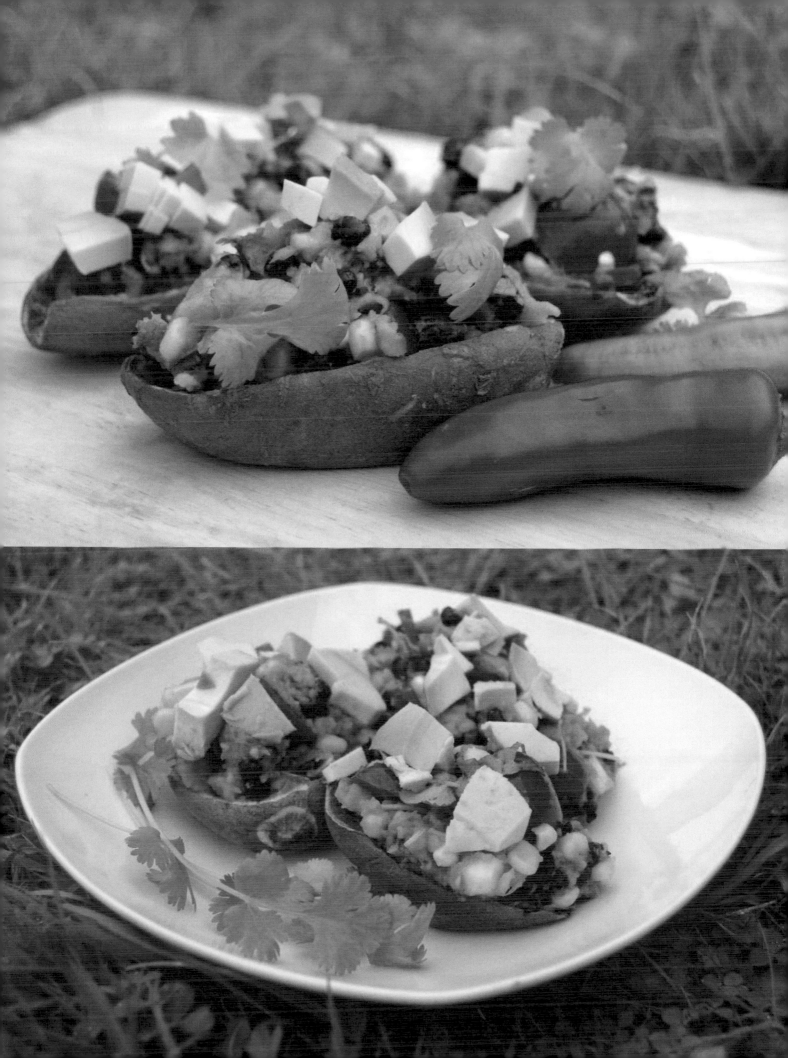

Sunflower Seed Cheese and Tomato Potato Bake

Serves 6 | 1h 25 mins **nf**

Cheap and easy to make vegan cheese and tomato potato bake. Just what you want on a cold winter's day. Very little prep work is needed and the oven does all the hard work. Can be prepped in advance and then kept in the fridge and baked in the oven when you're ready to eat.

I couldn't decide if this should be called a vegan cheese potato bake or vegan Spanish tortilla. It's somewhere in the middle as the sunflower seed cheese goes a bit foamy like the egg in a Spanish omelette.

Ingredients

- 2 cups / 300g **Cherry tomatoes**, halved
- 1 **Onion**, peeled and sliced
- 1 **Red pepper,** seeds and stem removed, cut into strips
- 1 lb / 450g **White potatoes**, cut into slices

Equipment

- Oven
- Baking dish 8"

Sunflower Seed Cheese Sauce

- 2 cups / 280g **Sunflower seeds**
- 2-4 tbsp **Nutritional Yeast** (page 108),
- depending on how much you like the flavour
- 1 tsp **Yeast extract**
- 3 cloves of **Garlic**
- 1 tsp **Turmeric**
- ½ tsp **Cayenne pepper**
- 2 cups / 500ml **Water**

Method

1. Blend together all of the sunflower seed cheese sauce ingredients.
2. In a large baking dish place a layer of sliced potatoes, sprinkle in the onion pepper and cherry tomatoes.
3. Pour over one-third of the sunflower cheese sauce, trying to fill in the gaps in between.
4. Repeat steps 2-3 a couple of more times until the dish is full.
5. Bake in the middle of the oven for 75-90 minutes at 190 C / 375 F.
6. Test that the potato is cooked by sliding in a knife and remove from the oven when cooked.
7. If the potato is not cooked and the topping is golden then reduce the heat by a quarter, move to the bottom of the oven and continue to bake.
8. Enjoy as soon as it's cool enough to eat. It is however just as delicious cold the next day.

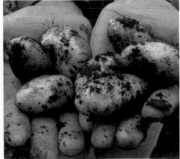

White Potatoes

The normal potato has been maligned in recent years, I did on the last page just declare it nutritionally inferior to sweet potatoes. However white potatoes are a great source of vitamin C, B6, fibre and potassium. The problem lies when they are cooked in oil. Enjoy them but not fried and do eat the skin as that's where lots of the goodness lies.

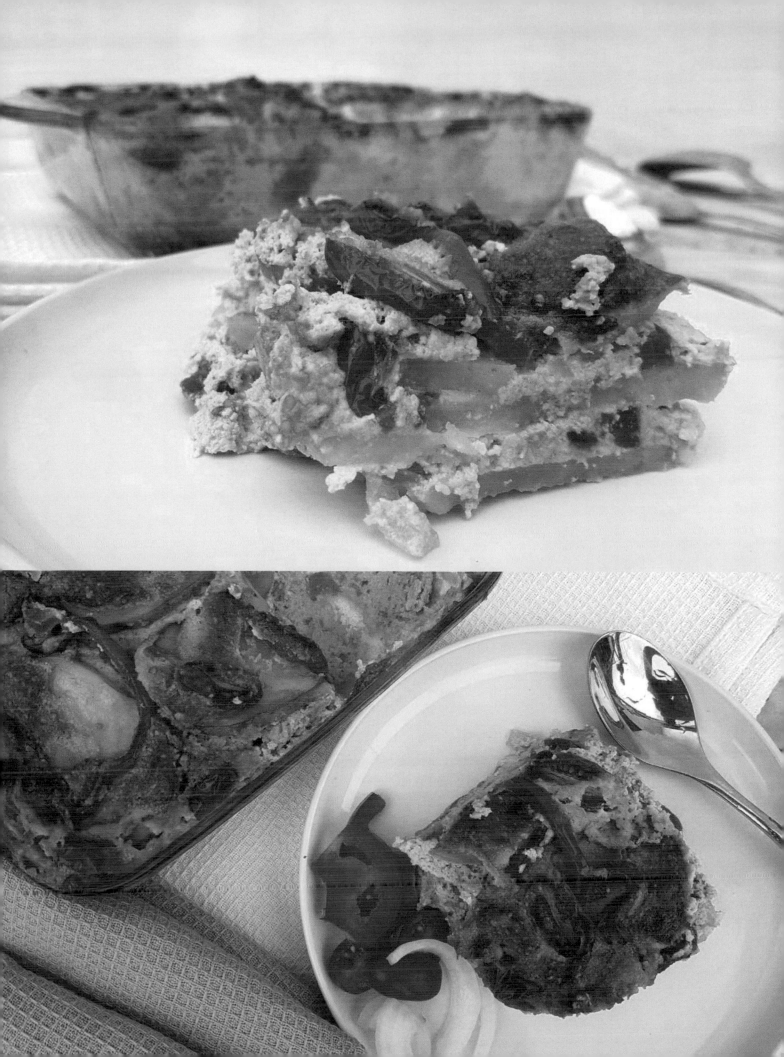

Roasted Cauliflower Cheese

Serves 6 | 1h 25 mins **nf**

This delicious roasted cauliflower cheese recipe uses butter beans to give a creamy and velvety texture. This means it's high in both protein and fibre. A great comfort recipe that is low in fat and free of oil.

The cauliflower is dry roasted to give a golden colour and a grilled taste. As no oil is used you need to keep a sharp eye on the oven when the cauliflower is roasting so it's taken out at exactly the right moment.

Ingredients

- 1 **Cauliflower**
- 1 can **Butter beans**
- 2 tbsp **Sesame seeds**
- 2 tbsp **Nutritional Yeast** (page 108)
- 1 clove **Garlic**
- ¼ tsp **Turmeric**
- 4 **Sun-dried tomatoes**
- 2 cups **Water**

Garnishes

- 1 cup **Cherry tomatoes**
- 1 tbsp **Chives**

Equipment

- Oven and Tray
- Blender

Method

1. Cut the stem off the cauliflower and break up into bite size florets.
2. Place these on a non stick tray and bake at 400°F / 200°C for about 20-25 minutes until the cauliflower starts to go golden brown.
3. Add the butter beans, sesame, garlic, turmeric, nutritional yeast sun-dried tomatoes and water to a blender and blend until smooth.
4. You may want to adjust the water in the cheese sauce depending on how thick/runny you like it.
5. Mix the roasted cauliflower with the cheese sauce and top with quartered cherry tomatoes and chives.
6. Broccoli works just as well in this recipe and I often make it with 50/50 Broccoli and Cauliflower.

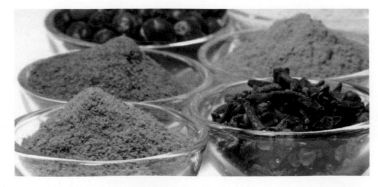

Inexpensive Spices

Spices can be expensive if bought from a supermarket in a little jar. I bulk buy 1k or 500g bags from wholesalers or Asian shops and decant into glass jars. Some are up to 90% cheaper than small jars and save packaging and running out every other week.

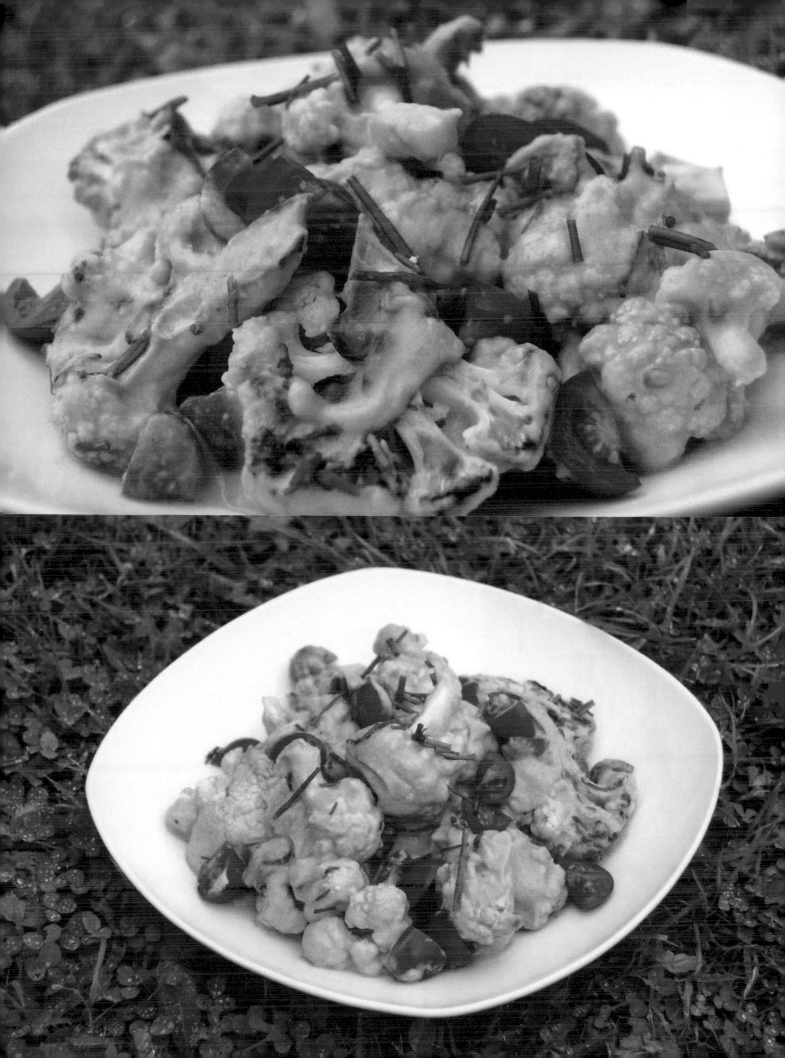

Creamy Tomato Courgette Spaghetti

Makes 2 main servings | 25 mins

This is an easy recipe for creamy tomato sauce with courgette spaghetti. The sauce is creamy thanks to the cashews and has no oil added. You can either steam the courgette spaghetti for 30 seconds or leave raw. In the summer I prefer the raw spaghetti and in the winter when I want something warmer I have the softer cooked version.

Ingredients

- 3 medium **Courgette / Zucchini**
- 1 cup / 150g **Cherry tomatoes**
- ½ cup / 75g **Cashews**
- 1 slice **Red onion**
- 1 clove **Garlic**
- 6 **Sun dried tomatoes**
- a pinch **Cayenne pepper**, depending on how spicy you like it

Optional Toppings

- Olives
- Basil leaves
- Tomatoes
- Nutritional Yeast (page 108)
- Macadamia or Pine nuts

Equipment

- Spiralizer
- Pan and Blender

Method

1. Cut the courgettes into spaghetti using your spiralizer / julienne slicer / vegetable peeler.
2. Steam or leave raw.
3. To steam just boil a few tablespoons of water and stir the courgette for about 30 seconds. Only a tiny amount of water is needed as once the courgettes heat up they release water.
4. You can just eat raw, leave as is / massage in some salt or dehydrate at a low temperature to soften the courgette.
5. Blend together all of the other ingredients until smooth to make the sauce.
6. Mix the sauce and spaghetti together.
7. Top with anything such as olives, basil, chopped tomatoes and eat within 3 days.

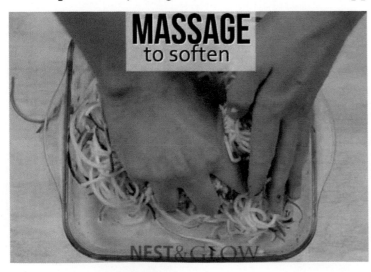

MASSAGE to soften

Video Recipes

If you are unsure about anything there is a video for every recipe in this book. All are about a minute long and show how to make the recipe clearly and concisely.

Find the video and full recipe at nestandglow.com by clicking on the category or searching.

Some recipes are book first exclusives, but all will be released on the site in due time.

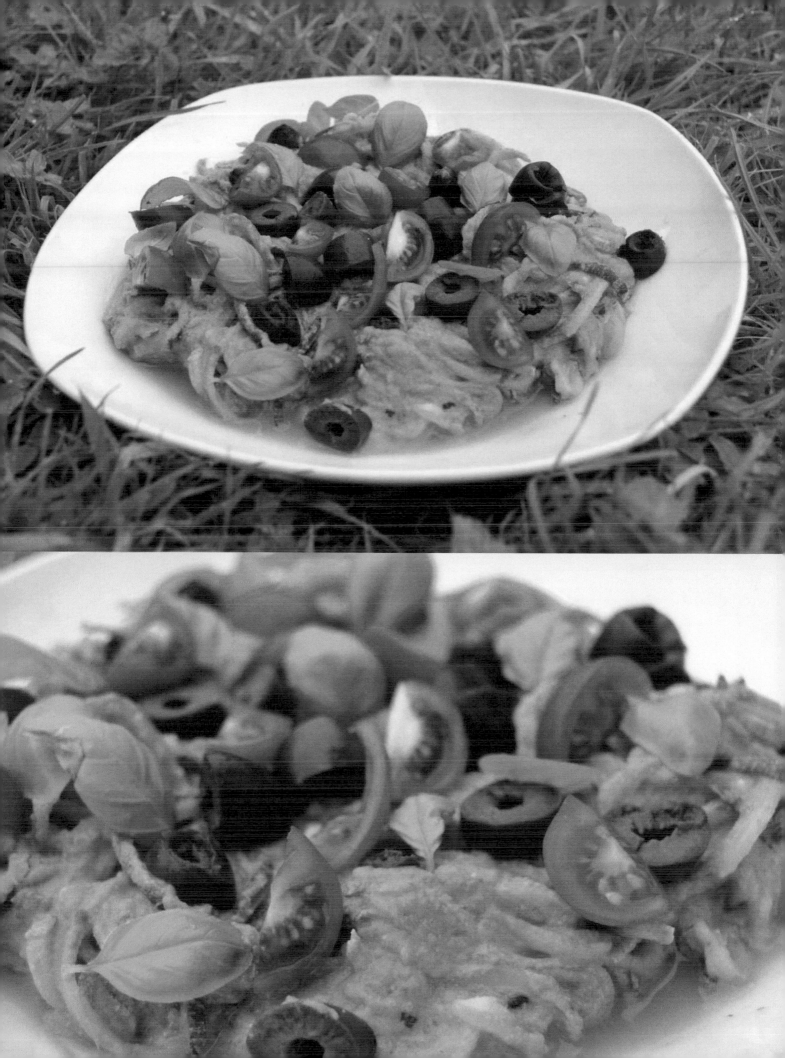

Chilli Stuffed Courgettes with Cashew Cheese

Makes 12 courgette halves | Serves 3 as a main | 25 mins

These chilli stuffed courgettes are a complete meal and easier to make than they look. They are topped with a homemade vegan cashew cheese. The chilli on its own is great, but stuffing inside courgettes and topping with a cashew cheese really makes this an impressive dish.

Ingredients

- 6 whole **Courgettes**

Chilli Ingredients

- 1 can chopped **Tomatoes**
- 1 can **Kidney beans**
- 1 **Onion**, diced
- 2 **Carrots**, diced
- 2 **Celery** stalks, diced
- 8 **Mushrooms**, sliced
- 2 tsp **Chilli powder**, adjust to taste
- 1 tsp **Cumin**
- 1 tsp **Turmeric**
- **Salt** and **Pepper** to taste

Cashew Cheese

- ⅓ cup / 50g **Cashews**
- 2 tbsp **Nutritional Yeast** (page 108)
- 1 clove **Garlic**
- 1 cup / 240ml **Water**
- pinch of **Salt**
- 2 tbsp **Tapioca** or Corn starch

Equipment

- Blender and Pan
- Oven and Tray

Method

1. Pre heat the oven to 350F / 180C.
2. Place everything for the chilli into a pan and simmer for 10 minutes with the lid on.
3. Cut the courgettes in half and leave the ends on – cut them symmetrically so that they lay flat.
4. Scoop out the flesh using a spoon, this can be used in soups or stews.
5. Fill the courgettes with the chilli.
6. Blend all of the cashew cheese ingredients together then simmer for 2-3 minutes until thick.
7. Pour on the cashew cheese and bake for 20 minutes until golden.

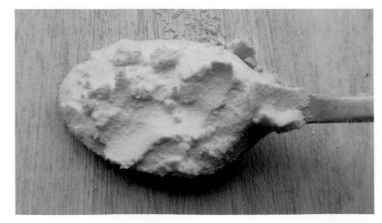

Tapioca Starch

Tapioca starch / flour is extracted from cassava roots and is gluten-free, grain-free, seed-free, nut-free and very low in sugar.

It has a mild taste and is very useful in gluten-free cooking in order to thicken or bind.

I use tapioca to give nut / seed mixes a stringy texture or to thicken coconut yoghurt.

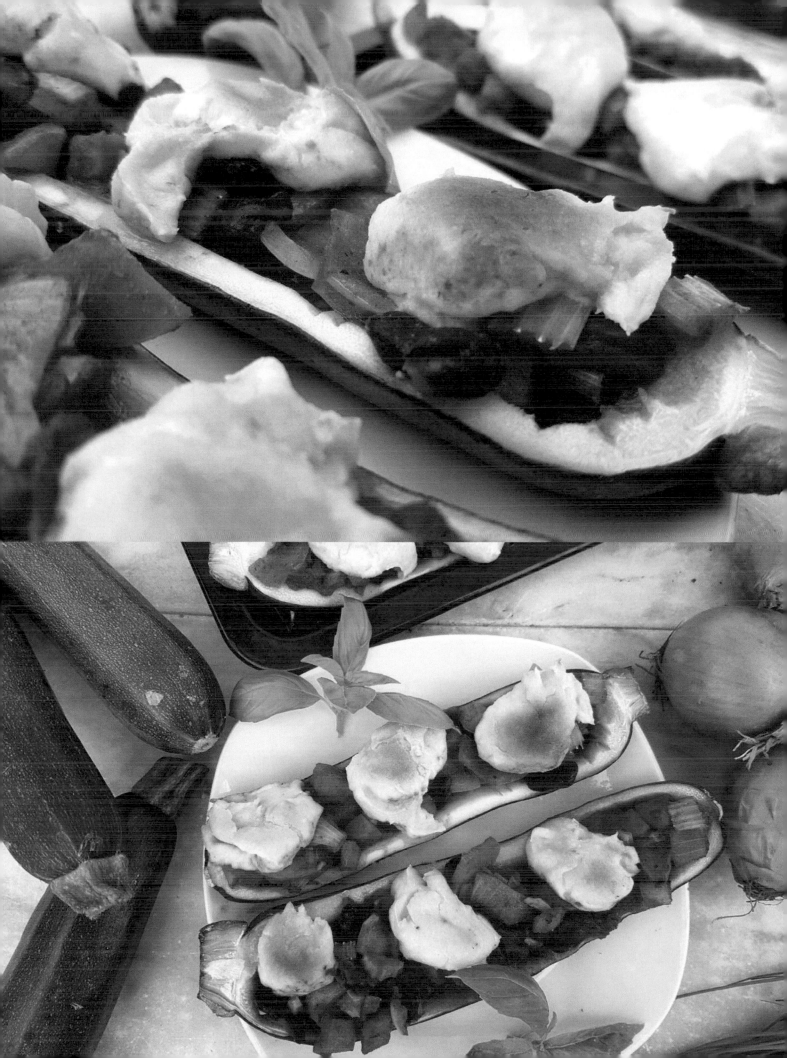

Seed Milks

Makes 2 pints per recipe | 15 mins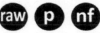

Making your own seed milk is inexpensive and much more nutritious than shop bought nut / seed milk. Once you start making your own you will never buy shop bought again.

Sunflower Vanilla Milk

- 1 cup / 140g **Sunflower seeds**
- 3 cups / 700ml **Water**
- 2 tbsp **Sweetener**, like maple syrup (optional)
- 1 tsp **Vanilla**
- a pinch of **Salt**

Sesame Cinnamon Milk

- 1 cup / 130g **Sesame seeds**
- 3 cups / 700ml **Water**
- 3-6 **Dates**, pitted
- 1 tsp **Cinnamon**
- 1 tsp **Vanilla**
- a pinch of **Salt**

Equipment

- Blender
- Nut milk bag / sieve / cheesecloth

Pumpkin Carrot Milk

- 1 cup / 130g **Pumpkin seeds**
- 3 cups / 700ml **Water**
- 2 **Carrots**
- 1" **Ginger**
- 1 tbsp **Cinnamon**
- 3-6 **Dates**
- a pinch of **Salt**

Hemp Cacao Milk

- 1 cup / 160g **Hemp seeds**
- 3 cups / 700ml **Water**
- 2 tbsp **Cacao / Cocoa powder**
- 3-6 **Dates**
- 1 tsb **Vanilla**
- a pinch of **Salt**

Sunflower, pumpkin and Sesame Method

1. Soak the seeds in water with a pinch of salt.
2. Leave for 8 hours or overnight then strain and rinse.
3. Add the seeds, water and all other ingredients apart from the vanilla, powders, or liquid sweeteners to a blender.
4. Blend on high for 2-3 minutes until all the seeds are finely ground.
5. Pour into a nylon milk bag / cheesecloth with a large bowl underneath.
6. Squeeze all of the moisture out.
7. Add the vanilla / cinnamon / maple syrup depending on the recipe and stir.
8. Enjoy the milk within 3 days. Keep in the fridge.
9. Use the fibre you are left with in baked goodies and smoothies.

Hemp Milk Method

- Place All into a blender and blend until smooth.
- Keep chilled and enjoy within 3 days.

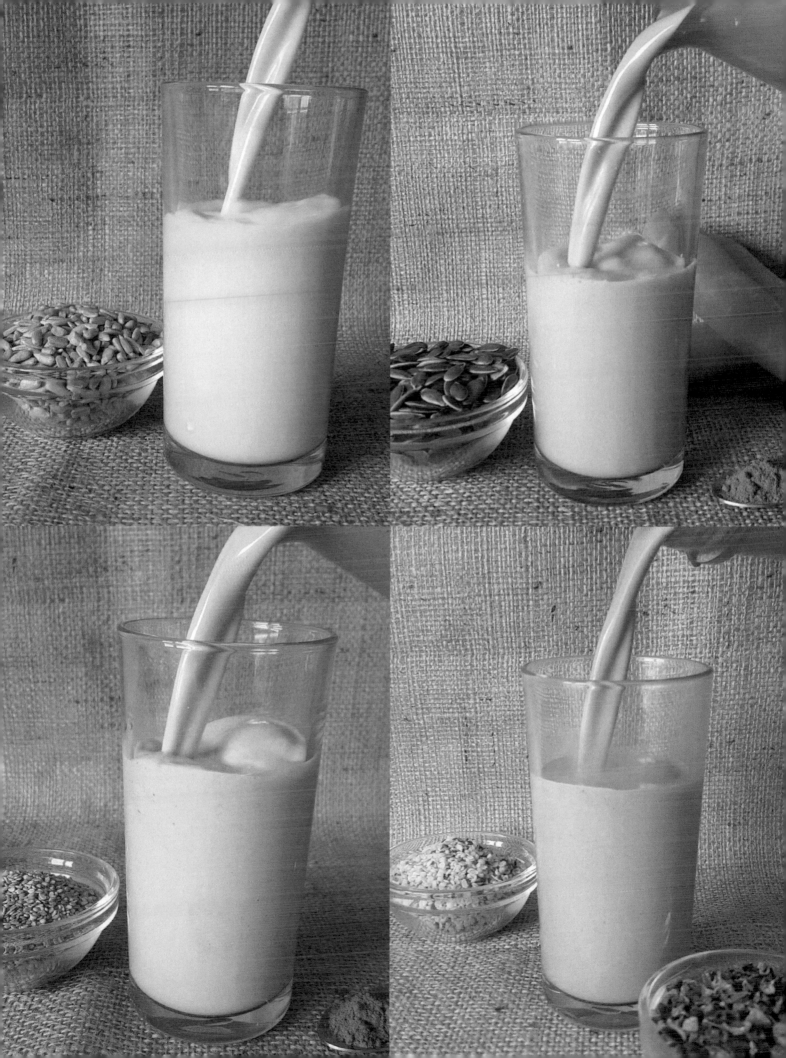

Fruit and Vegetable Shots

Makes single shot | 10 mins (raw) (p) (nf)

These easy to make fruit and vegetable shots can all be made quickly without a juicer. They are perfect for when you need a bit of a boost. The ingredients below are just a guideline and it's best to use produce that is local and in season. For the leafy greens I use greens growing wild in my garden such as nettles and dandelion leaves.

Leafy Greens Shot

- 1 **Lime**
- 1 handful **Leafy Greens** like Kale or Spinach
- 1 handful **Herbs** like Mint or Parsley
- 2 sticks **Celery**
- 1 **Kiwifruit**

Beetroot Lemon Shot

- 1 **Beetroot**, including tops if possible
- 1 **Apple**
- 1 **Lemon**, peeled

Carrot Turmeric Shot

- 3 **Carrots**
- 1 **Lemon**, peeled
- 1" **Ginger**
- ½ tsp **Turmeric**

Ginger Cayenne Shot

- 1 **Lemon**, peeled
- 4" **Ginger**
- pinch of **Cayenne pepper**
- a few tbsp **Water**

Equipment

- **Blender** and **Nut bag / Juicer**

Method

1. Peel the citrus fruit. Leave all other skin on for maximum nutrition.
2. Use a juicer and skip to step 6 or:
3. Place in a small jug blender and pulse until blended.
4. You may need to add some water to help blend.
5. Pour into a Nut Milk Bag (page 124) or cheesecloth and squeeze all the moisture out.
6. Enjoy the juice as soon as it's made as it will begin to degrade once juiced.
7. The pulp left over can be added into baked goodies such as cookies and pie crusts to partly substitute the oats or coconut flour.

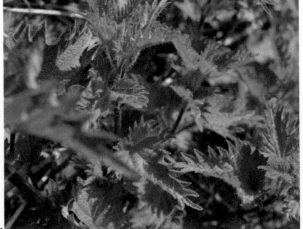

Wild Food

Wild food varies to farm-grown food as it has to survive on its own, often growing deep roots to reach nutrients. Commercially grown food is well cared with water and nutrients and doesn't have to struggle. Commercial produce is often varieties that are selected for shelf-life and how well they transport rather than nutrition or taste. I try to include wild food in my diet as it's free and has a different nutrient and vitamin profile to farmed foods.

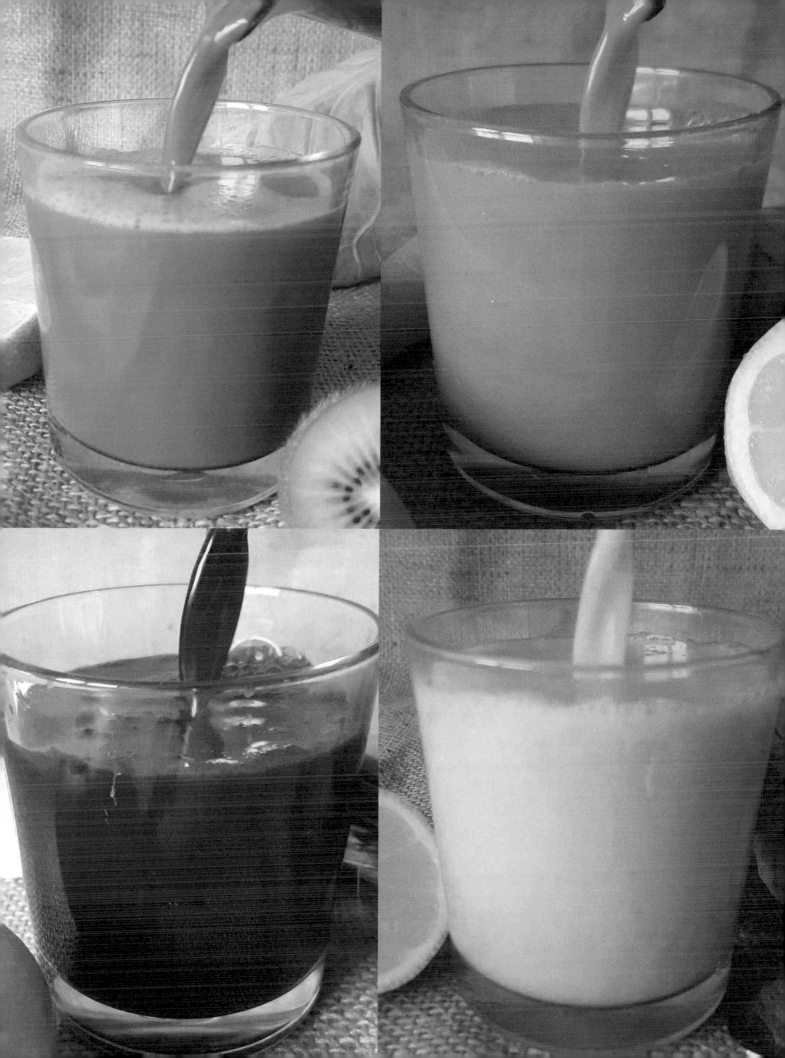

Golden Cashew Turmeric Milk

Makes 2 mugs| 10 mins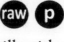

Spiced golden cashew milk with turmeric, ginger, cloves, black pepper, ginger and cinnamon. Easy to make and no pan is needed – just blend everything together and then pour over hot water and enjoy!

Ingredients

- 2 tbsp **Cashew nuts**
- 1 tbsp **Dates**
- 1 slice of **Ginger**
- ¼ tsp **Black pepper**
- ¼ tsp **Ground cloves**
- 1 tsp **Turmeric**
- ½ tsp **Cinnamon**
- ½ cup / 120ml **Water**
- 1 cup / 240ml **Hot water**

Equipment

- Blender
- Kettle

Method

1. Put everything apart from the hot water into a blender. Make sure that the dates have no stones in.
2. Blend for a few minutes, the dates take a while to break down.
3. Pour into a serving glass and top up with hot water – about a 1:1 ratio.
4. Enjoy straight away.
5. As this makes enough mix for two servings you can store the mix in the fridge for a few days.

Raw Hot Chocolate

Makes 2 mugs | 10 mins (raw) (p)

There is nothing like a hot creamy cup of hot chocolate for when you need a bit of winter comfort. If you're following a raw diet then make with water boiled that has cooled for 10 minutes.

Ingredients

- 2 tbsp **Cashews**
- 1 tbsp **Dates**, pitted
- 1 tbsp **Cacao / Cocoa powder**
- ½ cup / 120ml **Water**
- 1 cup / 240ml **Hot water**

Method

1. Blend together everything apart from the hot water in a small blender jug.
2. When this is smooth pour into your serving glass.
3. Pour over boiled water and enjoy this drink immediately.
4. You can keep the raw hot chocolate paste in the fridge for a few days and pour hot water on top when you're ready to enjoy.

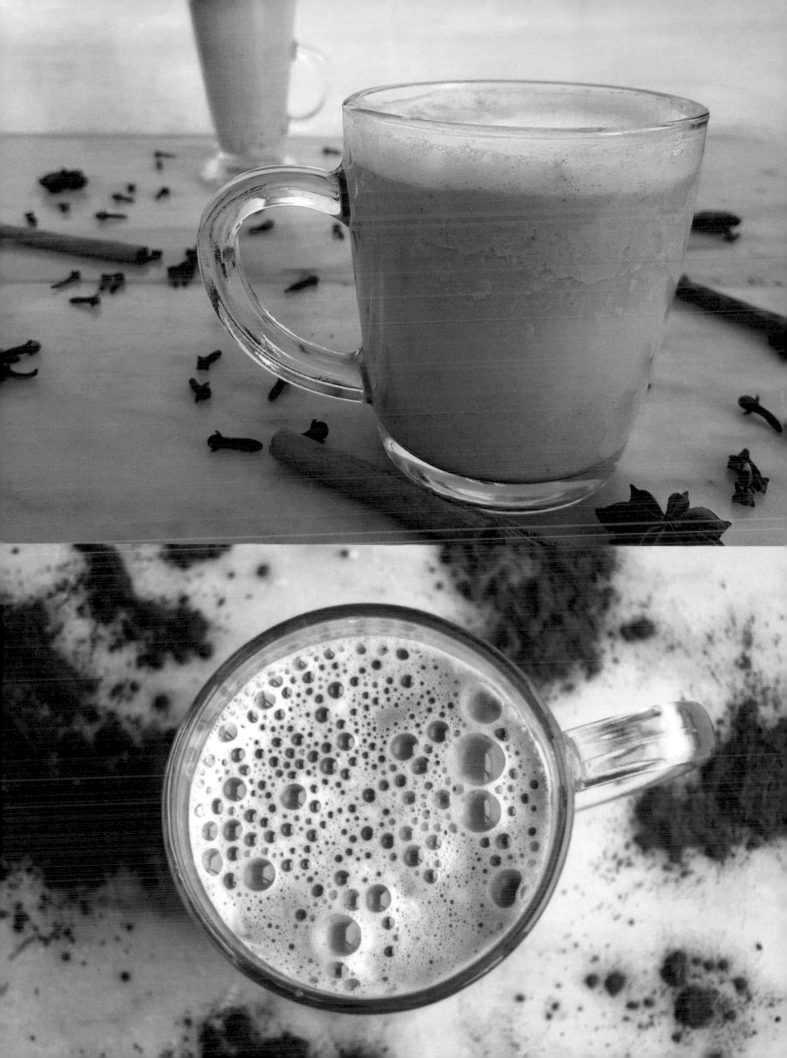

Index

Thank You

This book is the accumulation of over 30 years as a vegan and of those 15 years eating nutrient-dense plant-based foods. I've spent the last 2 years full time creating new recipes to inspire people to eat natural and unrefined foods high in nutrients and this book is a collection of the best.

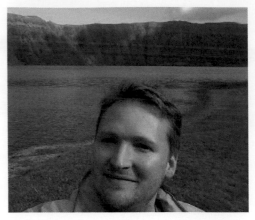

Huge thanks to the supporters of this project;

Andrew Johnson, Ágnes Borka, Alejandra Zamora, Ana Saveska, Andre Stanton, Anjuii James-Sawyers, Anna Te Rei, Audrey McBride, Beverly Aviani, Cassandra Voigt, Charlotte Ackerman, Christine Malek, Connie Drost, Craig Peterson, Cynthia de la Peña, Davide Sias, Debbie Ross, Desislava Nedyalkova, Diona Teh, Dovydas Se, Gaby Reyes Retana, Henry Bond, Ilca Andrikis, Joëlle Arseneau, Julie Mihalisin, Kate Newton, Kelly Parnell, Ladan Golshanara, Loma Naser, Lou Kats, Mary Laing, Megan Sinsley, Mônica Terezinha de Souza, Muhammad Nadhir Abdul, Olagoke Oluwatobiloba, Pierre-Olivier Teissier-Clément, Politou Maria, Rachel Emily, Riko Yano, Sheila Bond, Shima Jayasinghe, Sou Mônica, Stephanie D Jones, Teresa Murphy, Sunčica Milanović, Suzie Lewis

Links

- For more photos / videos / information and the latest recipes see nestandglow.com
- Follow my company for plant-based / natural content on social media @nestandglow
- Follow me on social media @bastiandurward

Thanks for purchasing this book, I hope you find a few recipes you love that become a regular part of your diet.

Thanks to all that have liked and shared my recipes online

NEST&GLOW